Fat *to* Fearless

Enjoy Permanent Weight Loss and
End Emotional Eating...For Good!

ASHER
FOX
C.Ht., Sc.B.

This book is dedicated to my parents, Otis and Lola, and the love they shared for each other. Although my father is no longer with us, his legacy and lessons continue to inspire me to be a better man.

And to Jonathan and Michael Dorn, without whose support on so many levels this book would not be in your hands. A man can live a lifetime and never be fortunate enough to find friends and brothers such as these.

A PERSONAL THANK YOU

The past couple of years have been transformational ones in my life. I've reached many milestones and seen several life-long dreams come true. I know that no man is an island, and the foundation of my success is the relationships I have forged with mentors from years past, as well as those who have come into my life more recently as teachers, advisors, and guides. I would like to publically acknowledge and thank those, without whose influence, I wouldn't be where I am today.

While my work now deals with root emotional and psychological causes, the foundation of my expertise in weight loss began in the health and fitness industry. Without the influences of these industry greats, much of my work and the thousands of client success stories that followed may never have happened.

I learned much from working with and observing Geoff Dyer. Both in his capacity in leading one of the country's top health club chains as well as president of IHRSA, the world's most prominent and influential fitness association with thousands of member fitness clubs, I observed how one man can influence the course of an entire industry through vision and leadership.

I will always treasure my time working with and learning from Merrill Brick. During our years together at the Orlando Fitness & Racquet Club, I came to know Merrill as a consummate professional and good friend, yet it has been his constant dedication to personal growth and improvement that has inspired me to adopt that same mission in my own life. Merrill continues to be one of the finest people I've ever known.

Victor Brick demonstrated to me the importance of being an industry trendsetter. By observing and listening to many of the stories of his early days in the industry, Victor Brick, CEO of Brick Bodies, as well as a leader with Planet Fitness, taught me the importance of taking risks and being willing to lead based on faith in yourself and a strong intuition about the future of your chosen field.

What I learned from Andrew Levine, one of my earliest mentors, has served as much of the foundation upon which I've built my own business success as well as consulted dozens of other entrepreneurs. I've personally watched him combine his almost endless knowledge of the fitness industry with an unmatchable work ethic to move virtual mountains to achieve success for both himself and his organization. Andrew's persistence and passion continues to inspire me.

CONTENTS

PART III
YOUR BELIEFS AND YOUR BODY

PART IV
NEW BODY BELIEFS

PART I

THE BEGINNING

INTRODUCTION

I can't believe it happened again! After working so hard, dieting, working out, being so aware of how much better I felt when I was at a healthy weight than when I was carrying extra body fat, I still managed to gain back all the weight in six weeks that I had lost over the prior three months. This time I gained the weight back so quickly, with so much in my professional life riding on my appearance, that I was still in a state of shock that I had allowed this to happen.

I had started my dieting and exercise knowing I needed to lose weight for an upcoming video shoot for my fitness business. Looking my best was integral to the success of a marketing campaign in which these videos played a central role. Five months out, I began the transformation process and in three months lost over 30 pounds. But then, with only two months left until the deadline to shoot the videos, I had regained the weight. I can't even describe how bad I felt as a fitness trainer, knowing that in two weeks I would be on camera for the world to see and over 40 pounds overweight. And this was not the first time I had done this; it was a cycle I was very familiar with.

The world is searching for "the next great diet" and "the next great fitness plan" that will finally allow all overweight people to once and for all shed their excess pounds. Eighteen years of clinical experience in working with weight loss clients, as well as over thirty years of personal experience with my own body, has taught me that this magic product and plan will never come. That is because the answer has far less to do with our knowledge of nutrition and exercise than it has to do with our deeply held subconscious beliefs about who we are, what we deserve, and what seems to be a lifetime of reinforcing experiences.

One of the most profound things I ever heard was from a client that had a life-long history of gaining and re-losing approximately 100 pounds several times in his life. He said, "If you want to know anything about diet or exercise, ask an overweight person. We have read it all, tried it all, researched it all, and it all worked for a time—until we regained the weight. We are experts."

Think about it. We live in the information age, but if information about nutrition and exercise were the key to permanent weight loss, everyone would have the bodies they want.

I have worked with several medical doctors, weight loss clinics, personal trainers, and health clubs over the years who began referring their patients, clients, and members to me when they just could not figure out why those who were having so much success would quit in the middle of their programs and regain their weight. By their way of thinking, they could understand people quitting if they were not getting results, but often it seemed to be those who were getting the best results that would stop showing up for their appointments and ultimately disappear, only to resurface at the clinic or health club a year later weighing more than they did when they had started originally.

The doctors, fitness, and weight loss professionals also suffered from the same false premise that current results, those produced from a good nutrition and exercise program alone, lead to long-term success. But for the countless millions who have experienced changing their behavior and losing weight only to go back to their old habits and regain their weight, nothing could be further from the truth.

What if the truth is closer to the opposite? What if losing the weight actually triggers something deep in our subconscious that directly leads to our own self-sabotage? What if the same parts of our hidden psyche, often hidden since childhood, is what has caused us to be overweight our entire lives? What if our subconscious is not happy to sit idly by while we consciously decide to change our bodies, something that determines so much about what we experience in our daily lives? From thousands of clients over almost 20 years, and a lifetime of personal experience, I know this to be true.

This book is about understanding the "why" behind the questions of your life-long struggle with weight. It is about understanding that the shape of your body, which often dramatically affects the shape of your life in ways you do not yet understand—but soon will—is about your thoughts, emotions, and subconscious beliefs.

Do you need to live a healthy lifestyle consisting of a good nutrition plan with an appropriate amount of activity? Yes, but it is our thoughts and feelings that determine our willingness to do that, to not use food to satisfy our emotions.

While most people who have struggled with lifelong weight issues know to some degree that they often eat for emotional reasons, that is only the tip of the iceberg. This book is about transformation at the deepest levels that leads to the changes that so many people have sought for a lifetime.

Will you uncover the hidden secrets to lifelong weight loss and find the tools to finally transform your body in a truly lasting way? Yes. But my promise to you is that when this journey is over, as wonderful as that will be, you will have found something much greater. You will have found a degree of happiness, peace, and self-love like you have never known. I have, and I know you will as you make the journey from *Fat to Fearless*®.

~ Asher Fox

THE ASHER FOX STORY

Life can be challenging for a 300-pound personal trainer, trust me, I know. Not all of my years in the fitness industry were spent being so overweight, but they were all spent on the roller coaster of weight loss ups and downs that came with constantly losing weight only to regain it.

I only reached a full 300 pounds once in my career, and I didn't stay that heavy for very long. On average, however, I was always struggling with at least an extra 50 pounds. I was the poster child for "knowledge doesn't equal success."

I was also the poster child for "desire itself does not create success." In my entire life there was nothing I desired with more intensity than the body I saw many of my fitness colleagues have, which they appeared to obtain with ease.

I entered the fitness industry and became a certified personal trainer with the belief that knowing so much about fitness, being surrounded by fit people constantly, and having my very income and livelihood depend on my body would guarantee I would look and feel the way I wanted. But in the end, I found that I still struggled with the same issues I always had. Food was not my friend and having to exercise often felt like my enemy.

I had grown up as an overweight child in a predominately overweight family. Both of my parents had weight issues and my household was anything but a model for healthy eating habits. My parents moved a lot when I was a child. My dad liked Florida and my mom wanted to live in Virginia, so we lived in both, with several compromises in between.

As a child, this was a rather lonely life. We rarely lived anywhere longer than a year or so, and that didn't present many options to create lasting friendships. I had a brother and a sister, but both were more than 15 years older than me and had already left home and started their own families.

I turned to fiction for friendship. I spent time with Superman, Batman, Spiderman and other comic book heroes. While I learned lessons from those books about right and wrong and good overcoming evil, which mirrored the lessons I learned from my father, I also learned what a hero, what "good" looked like. He was muscular, fit, and always inspired admiration from the female characters. I learned that "good" didn't look like me.

As I grew older, I also learned that I liked more than food. I liked girls. A lot. This was mostly a one-way obsession that was the first of many lessons I learned about how my weight and body seemed to limit my happiness in the areas I wanted most. It wouldn't be the last. The inferiority complex that developed around my appearance and my weight bled over into other areas of my life, and I soon found myself always assuming that I would be picked last no matter what the activity or social venue.

For some reason, despite being overweight and considered less than attractive at the time, I set my sights high. I was always attracted to and pursued the most beautiful girls in school, the girls who very much liked the athletic, fit, good-looking guy that I didn't seem to be.

On the surface, this would seem to be fools folly, yet years later I came to understand pursuing women that would reject me was subconsciously driven, like many of my self-sabotaging behaviors, in order to prove to myself what I really believed: I simply wasn't good enough.

Throughout high school, I never had a girlfriend and had a very limited social life. Friday nights and weekends were spent mostly at the local movie theater with the less than "in" crowd.

I believed my weight was the primary issue that kept me from getting the girls I thought I wanted and living the "popular life."

Throughout those teenage years, I went on many diets and fitness programs in an attempt to solve my weight problem. Sometimes I had success and sometimes I didn't. No matter how much weight I lost, my social status and the way I felt about myself in the long run never really changed. Inevitably, I always regained the weight.

All of this began to shift and change shortly after high school. An auto accident when I was younger left me with sudden back pain at 18 that led to almost complete paralysis from the waist down in a very short period of time. Surgery was the only answer. After a major operation to repair my back, I began the process of learning to walk again. I knew it was time for significant change in my life, and as I prepared to move to college, I decided on a new career path that I believed would simultaneously take care of my three major issues. I decided the best way to fix my weight issues, lack of social success with women and the "in" crowd, as well as begin to repair my flagging self-esteem was to become a certified personal trainer. Besides, what else could you do to financially put yourself through college that also seemed to have so many great perks?

I trained hard and I worked hard and soon had my fitness credentials. While I didn't have the body I wanted, I lost the vast majority of the weight and was a good solid average. What I lacked in that beach body physique, I made up through hard work and great people skills. From the beginning, I understood the weight loss struggles of the masses and created fitness programs that strongly resonated with the hopes and dreams and deepest fears of those who had grown up overweight.

At the age of 22, starting with only $300 left from a student loan, I built one of the largest personal training businesses in the state of Florida. I had three locations in Tallahassee, multiple trainers, and a dream to take over the fitness world. Yet I still struggled with my own weight.

I believed I was helping people to recover from how I used to be, but the truth was that I was barely treading water myself while I tried to throw them a life raft. I was a walking encyclopedia of fitness knowledge and had more than six certifications, including Medical Exercise Specialist, the highest level of certification available in the industry at the time.

Yet all of this knowledge didn't truly change me or make it easier for me to do the "right" things. I still loved to eat, I still used food to make me feel better, my own workouts were far and few between, and my nights were still spent alone. I had changed my outside, but I had not changed my inside.

Despite frequent and large fluctuations in my own weight, my clientele continued to grow. Only later would I realize that by training with me they didn't feel the judgment and pressure they put on themselves with other trainers whose bodies reflected the fitness stereotype. My own body was enabling them to justify their slower progress. Some were experiencing weight loss success while training with me, while others struggled to move the scale despite my best efforts and complete dedication to their success.

Even at this point, early in my career, the therapist that I was to become began to notice the differences between those who succeeded and those who didn't. The ones who either experienced no weight loss at all, or quickly regained the lost weight after stopping their training, needed something more than what personal training and a good nutrition program could provide. I wanted to give "that" to them, whatever "it" was. I also wanted to give it to myself.

I was 14 when I first read *Unlimited Power* by Anthony Robbins. I was captivated by the idea that the vast majority of people were only using a fraction of their available mental power and that there were proven methods to tap into more of our potential. I was entranced by the thought of what was possible by learning to apply the techniques in the book.

Much of Anthony's work was founded on the principles of Neuro-Linguistic Programming (NLP), a way of learning to structure your thoughts and internal processes to change your inner experiences and outer results. Many years later I would train with Richard Bandler, the co-founder/creator and driving force behind the development of NLP. When I realized my clients needed more than fitness training and nutrition coaching to be successful, I decided that renewing my study of NLP and learning hypnosis would be my first steps to finding new solutions for my clients' old problems. Hopefully I would get the answers for me as well.

I dedicated myself to learning everything there was to know about how to transform and change at the very deepest level of one's being. I knew that long-term success depended not only on a person losing weight and being fit, but also on feeling fit or thin or attractive or whatever it was that was important to them. They needed to be "it," not simply pursue "it" with the goal of having "it." As long as it was something they were chasing, it was something outside of themselves that they would never catch.

I was determined to learn all that I needed to know to create programs that would help clients overcome their weight issues by overcoming the limiting beliefs that trapped them in their overweight bodies. These new protocols were unheard of in the industry and would launch my career to new heights while finally giving me the tools to truly help people in a lasting way. Fate, or my subconscious as I have learned to call it, had different plans for my immediate future.

In December 1997, my father was unexpectedly diagnosed with terminal liver cancer. On February 25, 1998, the greatest man I have ever known passed away and my life changed. For years I had worked 7 days a week, 12 to 16 hours a day, trying to be what in my mind was a success. While I now know much of that was driven by low self-esteem pushing me to prove to the world that I had value, much of it was also driven by my desire to financially provide for my parents the things they never had. With my father gone, and the insurance he left behind taking care of my mother, much of my motivation to work so hard evaporated overnight. I began to view my priorities and life very differently.

It suddenly seemed to matter far less how many locations my personal training business had or how much money I was making or was going to make in the future as we franchised our fitness studios. The number of hours I was working seemed absurd in relationship to the cost of living the life of loneliness that had become my home.

While not realizing it before, after my father's death it became apparent that he was who held our family together. That year, I spent my first Thanksgiving alone without family. I felt empty and abandoned, alone in my townhouse eating Thanksgiving dinner in the form of a burrito from the local gas station. I had hit emotional rock bottom and my weight began to balloon up and out of control.

Finding someone to spend my life with *now*, instead of in the *future* after attaining the financial success to be able to provide for a family, became my number one goal.

I can't say that I consciously changed much in my life; the only noticeable outward difference was my complete lack of enthusiasm for work. Yet my heartache and the loneliness I felt must have reached out in a way it hadn't before. Within six months, I met the girl who I believed had walked into my life straight from my dreams. Between my loneliness and the amazement that for the first time a woman this intelligent, funny, and beautiful actually wanted me, I fell in love quickly. She had just left a long-term relationship and her recent breakup fueled her need to ease her own loneliness and feelings of abandonment as well. The relationship progressed very quickly.

What I thought would be a fairytale turned out to more closely resemble a Wikipedia article on the effects of low self-esteem on a relationship. Both of us brought our own baggage, but for me, this relationship seemed to prove what I had always feared about myself. I was second best, not good enough, unlovable, and in some unchangeably innate way—flawed.

I know now this had far less to do with her or any actual events that took place in the relationship, and everything to do with the subconscious beliefs I had about myself. By the time the relationship ended, I weighed almost 300 pounds and my inattention, lack of enthusiasm, and the constant emotional upheaval of my relationship had led to the demise of my business as well.

To make matters worse, my extreme weight gain had put too much pressure on my back and within a month of our breakup I couldn't walk again and needed another back surgery to avoid paralysis. Having lost everything, my mother came and collected me from the city where only a couple of years earlier I had been such a success, a fixture in the community, constantly appearing on local radio and TV espousing the virtue of fitness and good nutrition, and took me and my shattered body home for another surgery and to heal. I was determined that I would come back stronger than before.

Almost a year to the day that I left, barely able to walk and weighing over 300 pounds, I returned with the body I had spent a lifetime trying to achieve. To this day my friends laugh about it. I drove into town a seemingly changed man. I was lean, muscular, energetic, and somehow racing stripes had found their way onto my convertible Mustang. With the help of my hairstylist friend, my hair had gone from dark brown to blonde. I thought I had done it. I thought I was cool. I had conquered my body demons and this was going to be my time to shine!

It wasn't my time to shine. Within six months, I gained 50 pounds, and over the next couple of years I added another 50. Intermixed with the weight loss roller coaster were ups and downs in relationships too numerous to mention. Some were good, others were bad, and none of them filled my void the way food did. It would take another 10 years of hard life lessons and dedicating myself to understanding the psychological, behavioral, and motivational reasons behind my chronic inability to lose weight before I ever saw that fit, muscular, lean body again.

The breaking point for me came when I had a relationship with a young woman who seemed to be my dream come true. At this point you probably realize that I thought this a lot. I had accumulated a lot of education and many credentials over the years and was a Clinical Hypnotherapist and Hypnotherapy instructor at the time I met her.

I believed that I had resolved most of my own issues, and while I went into the relationship knowing she had a lot of emotional healing to do, I thought that since I was a well-respected healing professional, I could provide her with the resources to heal and referrals to other therapists while encouraging her through the process. This was wishful thinking, and I now know it was a reflection of my unhealed and subconscious need to feel better about myself by helping someone else. It was projection at its worst.

The next several months were undoubtedly the most miserable time of my life. Her issues were far more extreme than I had ever imagined, culminating in her diagnosis of a significant personality disorder. Her pathological lying, emotional mood swings, insecure need to criticize my body, suicide threats, and eventual infidelity resurrected demons in myself that I thought were long gone.

Finally, in an emotional night where her most recent and worst set of lies and infidelity were revealed, the relationship ended. As painful as it was, I had never felt such relief. I knew I had allowed this to happen as a result of my own deep subconscious belief that I didn't deserve any better. I'm sure you aren't surprised to hear that I was also fat again.

I couldn't believe that with all of my credentials, training, background, and knowledge, that I could let someone like this into my life. I couldn't believe I had gained weight again. I knew that whatever was inside me that was still unhealed was responsible for both, as well as every other act of self-sabotage in all other areas of my life.

This time there would be no stopping me. My life became about finding the missing pieces of the puzzle to finally heal myself and others. I would have true high self-esteem. I would love myself and not accept unloving people into my life. And yes, I would finally get the body I wanted and keep it. As countless weight loss clients I have had since that time can tell you, that is exactly what I did.

Looking back, perhaps it could not have happened any other way for me to learn these lessons to bring the *Fat to Fearless*® program to you now. I needed to have those ups and downs to begin to see the patterns and trends that are at the heart of life-long weight loss issues. I needed to learn firsthand that I didn't feel bad about myself because I was overweight, but was overweight because I felt bad about myself at a deeper level, far beneath my conscious awareness. Being overweight, bad relationships, financial self-sabotage—these were all symptoms with one common cause rooted in my subconscious.

Over the 18-year journey that it took for me to achieve and keep the body I now have, I have become a successful Subconscious Behaviorist, Clinical Hypnotherapist and Hypnotherapy instructor, a Certified Master Life Coach and life coaching instructor, a licensed Master Practitioner of Neuro-Linguistic Programming and an NLP Trainer, a Cognitive Behavioral Coach, a Certified Relationship Coach, an EFT Practitioner, an author, a radio show host and public speaker, and have been on the faculty of two institutions teaching the next generation of therapists and coaches. I learned a lot, but more importantly, I actively applied that knowledge to myself everyday. Now I am passing the baton to you.

In this book you will learn a lot about the power of the subconscious mind. You will uncover your deepest beliefs, some you may not even be aware of, and how they have affected your ability to lose weight. You will learn the way the mind works to create motivation and how not understanding that is a major factor in why very few ever reach their weight loss goals.

You will also come to understand what it takes to create long-term change instead of short-term results. You will finally find the answers to why you have struggled with weight issues most of your life. You will learn the connection those difficulties have to all areas of your life that you are dissatisfied with.

I believe my struggles were for a greater purpose: to share this book and this program with you, and to begin a new era of the way we approach the issue of losing weight. It's not about treating symptoms but curing causes. It is not about losing weight, but about gaining life. This work, my life's work, is what I now humbly offer to you.

It is time for you to go from *Fat to Fearless*®.

WHAT'S FEAR GOT TO DO WITH IT?

Many people have asked why this book and the program is titled *Fat to Fearless®*; specifically, they want to know what fear has to do with losing weight. After many years of working with clients around weight loss, I can tell you that anything we want to do but have repeatedly failed at, is in some way linked to fear.

For most people, especially when it comes to weight loss, this fear is subconscious. It is a fear of the unknown. What will life be like when I lose weight and keep it off? What if I do not deserve the life I want? What if I lose weight but my life doesn't change the way I think it will? These are just a few of the many subconscious fears that cause people to sabotage their weight loss success.

Beyond that, losing weight and living the life you want to live, in the healthy body you deserve, is an act of self-love. It's well known that fear is the antidote to love. This has been known since ancient times and spoken of in texts like the Bible where I John 4:18 says, "There is no fear in love. But perfect love drives out fear, because fear has to do with punishment. The one who fears is not made perfect in love."

This has also been understood in our modern times and has been applied in countless self-help programs. Weight loss is the one area where the role of fear is not understood well, but is critical to long-term success. If you are significantly overweight and feel as if you are less valuable as a human being in any way because of it, you do not truly love yourself to the degree that enables lifelong weight loss, and where there is no love there is always some degree of fear. Sometimes you are aware of the fear and sometimes it is subconscious. When something is subconscious it means, by definition, you may not even know or believe it exists.

As you go through the *Fat to Fearless*® program, you will find that whatever is in your subconscious that keeps you from loving yourself, and has caused you to always sabotage your weight loss efforts, probably found its beginning in the garden of fear. Bringing up those fears to overcome them is also why the word "fat" is in the title.

Some people might believe that my use of the word "fat" is insensitive, and they are right. I specifically use the word "fat" in the title and throughout the book because unlike more sensitively chosen words, "fat" often brings up a strong emotional response in people who have struggled with being overweight most of their lives. To heal something, we must feel it first. To overcome fear, we mustn't hide from our pain.

Like the verse quoted above from the Bible, fear has to do with punishment. Those who have suffered from the weight loss/weight gain cycle most of their lives know that there are not many punishments worse than hating your own body that you live in every minute of every day. To lose weight, you must learn to love yourself. To love yourself, you must eliminate the subconscious fears and blocks that are holding you back.

The good news is that with the *Fat to Fearless*® program, I will help you do this like I have so many others. Even better, the benefits of doing this work go beyond the transformation you experience in your body. When you eliminate the fears and subconscious blocks that have kept you overweight, you will find that these very same fears and blocks have been holding you back from fully expressing your potential in other areas of life as well. You find that you embrace and live life more fully, more authentically, and not just with a healthy body but also with an open heart. You will live life fearlessly.

IT'S NOT YOUR FAULT . . . YET!

In today's world of ready-made victims, finger-pointing, and avoidance of self-blame, it may seem self-serving to have one of the opening sections begin with the statement that "it's not your fault." After all, what more do we ever want to hear about any of our problems? If it's not our fault, it means there's nothing we could have done. We are absolved of responsibility. Yet not being our fault isn't the same as saying there was nothing we could've done, but what it may mean is that we didn't know what to do. **Then.**

This is the type of blamelessness that is absolving in an unsatisfying way, because it inherently implies that there is something that CAN be done now. It's the type of blamelessness that both absolves, while at the same time spurs us to action by taking away past excuses.

Perhaps there is no subject more neglected in schools than the most basic understanding of the way our mind works. Sure, we have some basic knowledge of what the conscious and subconscious minds are, and perhaps even a rudimentary understanding of how they work. It's a lot like much of the technology we use today. We certainly understand enough about iPods, computers, and DVD players to use them in our daily life, yet when they break or don't work as planned, how many of us can take them apart and bring them back to life? Not many of us.

Unlike our electronics, which can easily be repaired by a readily available local technician or even more easily replaced, when things go wrong in our life it's often not so easy to set things right again. That's because what happens in our life, and as you'll soon learn in our bodies, is a result of what happens in our minds. Unfortunately many of us would know more about the parts and pieces of our malfunctioning DVD player than we know about the mechanics of our own mental landscape.

While for most, the subconscious is nothing but an ambiguous word denoting mystery; for those of us who spend our lives studying it, we know that there are rules and truths that govern how it functions. This is good news, because invariably almost every result you have ever produced in your life in any area is a direct result of the activity of your subconscious mind. Nowhere is this truer than in our bodies. This is good news for those who've struggled their whole lives with trying to lose weight. It means that there is a reason outside of failed dieting attempts, supplements, and abandoned exercise programs as to why you've never been able to shed the pounds and keep them off. It also means that there is a solution.

Amidst the rules, truths, and science behind how the subconscious mind works is a proven path to changing it. Everything from your emotional cravings for food, to your lack of motivation around exercise, and your seemingly unavoidable fate to regain lost weight is rooted in your subconscious DNA.

Your subconscious DNA is the mental template that your unconscious mind, which controls your body's autonomic functions ranging from metabolism to the very regulation of your breath, uses to construct both your body and your life. To lose weight and keep it off requires changing this template and reinventing yourself from the inside out.

Many years ago, I took advantage of my time working in gyms and health clubs to begin to study the mindsets of those who had the bodies I always wanted. What made them different than me? Why after the end of a long day did I make the decision to skip my workout and go home while they stayed long after the gym closed, sculpting the bodies that I envied? Why, when it would often take every ounce of willpower I had to avoid that doughnut or pastry or even just that second serving I didn't need, did they easily turn away without seemingly a second thought? I had to know.

I realized that the answer wouldn't be found simply in their decisions related to nutrition and exercise because that answer was simple. They made the better choices that I didn't. I realized that the answer would be in examining their life from a broader perspective. I needed to know less about what they did on the outside and more about who they were on the inside.

Was it some superhuman willpower gene they were born with that unfortunately skipped over the weight-challenged masses? Perhaps they had been blessed with perfect childhoods, free of sugary temptations while surrounded by healthy role models. When I began my study I had the sense that the answer would be both simple and complex at the same time.

Over the years, first through observation and self-experimentation, then formal education, and finally the synthesis of all of these things, which resulted in my successful work with weight loss clients, I found the answer. Once the mystery was unraveled, I discovered that like all great mysteries there is nothing mysterious at all, just things previously unknown or misunderstood. Like a great treasure hidden in an ancient temple uncovered by an adventurous movie archaeologist, at the end of my search for the answer what stared back at me was "me." Specifically, my subconscious mind was revealed as the great architect of not only my prior weight loss failures, but it was also the subconscious minds that were attached to the owners of those bodies I coveted that had sculpted their enviable physiques.

I had found the secret to creating lifelong weight loss and building the body of my dreams. But unlike that archaeologist in the movie that after finding the great treasure has little to do until his next sequel, my work was just beginning. If you continue on through this book, you will find that yours is also.

This is meant as a bit of warning. Getting results isn't as simple as reading the words on these pages; it is going to take your participation and your effort. I'm telling you it will not be easy, but I'm also telling you it will be worth it. The great secret to permanent weight loss is that when you change your subconscious DNA to create the body you've always wanted, quite often the *life* you always wanted follows. Not because you're finally thin, but because you became on the inside the type of person who loves themselves enough to automatically and without effort make the choices that created that thinner and healthier body. Change doesn't happen in a vacuum and when you make those types of powerfully positive changes in one area of your life, you will carry those same habits of self-love and self-care, now etched into your subconscious, into other areas of your life as well.

If I didn't know how important losing weight is to you, I might feel a little guilty. I began this chapter by telling you it's not your fault, but I've already begun taking that blamelessness away. As I said, it wasn't your fault because you didn't know there was a better way. The minute you bought this book, that began to change. If you've read this far, you already have enough knowledge that if you choose not to go forward you are also choosing to accept the responsibility of being over-weight. From this moment forward, with each page you read and exercise you do, you are gaining knowledge, insight, and the ability to change yourself in a way that will lead to lasting weight loss, improved self-esteem, and the best possible ver-sion of yourself. From here forward, you only have yourself to blame if you choose to not follow through.

While this may seem like a scary concept for some, I've per-sonally always found it empowering. To accept responsibility also means to accept that I can create the outcome I want. It's all up to me, just as now it's all up to you.

Many times throughout this book, I reiterate the impor-tance of doing the exercises and engaging in the processes. As you will learn, repetition is one of the most powerful ways to influence the subconscious mind. The exercises in this book, as well as the Hypnotherapy Audio Sessions, are designed to work with both your conscious and subconscious minds in a way to produce lasting permanent change. Outside of personal sessions with me, this is certainly the fastest way to create these changes, but it doesn't happen overnight.

It's important as you do the work to be patient and loving with yourself. You are not a digital switch that can be changed in a blink or instant, but instead you are participating in a form of evolution that is fueled by internal experiences. Give yourself the time to have these experiences and work at your own pace. I trust you will know the difference between loving self-patience and self-sabotaging procrastination. While you may not yet fully trust yourself, I trust the "you" deep within your subconscious that is waiting for an opportunity to create the body and life you want and deserve.

If you choose to move forward, know that this is uncharted territory. You are moving forward into the world, taking full responsibility for the outcomes you create, both when it comes to weight loss and the rest of your life. I will be with you on this journey every step of the way, yet your journey, like mine was, will be uniquely yours.

WHAT IF I'M HAPPY BEING FAT?

There are those who would disagree with the idea that being overweight implies a lack of self-love. As a matter of fact, there are several blogs and websites dedicated to the idea that "big is beautiful" and you should accept and love yourself regardless of your weight. I couldn't agree more.

The purpose of the *Fat to Fearless*® program isn't to give everyone a fitness model body, but for you to have the body that's perfect for you once you've cleared away negative subconscious beliefs, false fears, negative self-judgments, and an overall lack of self-love. When this is done, it's very hard to be significantly overweight because of the pervading beliefs in our culture.

At the heart of the *Fat to Fearless*® program and at the foundation of my work as a Subconscious Behaviorist is the understanding that subconscious beliefs, many of which we are unaware of, play themselves out both in the circumstances we create in our lives and in our very bodies and physical health. For this reason, deep feelings of inadequacy, low self-esteem, not being good enough, and unworthiness frequently lead to self-sabotage in many areas of life, including losing weight and keeping it off. When you understand this, as you will by the time you finish this program, the only way to be able to have resolved negative beliefs about yourself and maintain the habits and behaviors that led to being significantly overweight is if you have absolutely, at a deep subconscious level, no correlation between physical attractiveness and self-worth, and in no way link being overweight with attractiveness. In our culture this is almost impossible to do.

Put more simply, as you will learn in this program, one of the core functions of the subconscious mind is to prove to you that your subconscious beliefs are true. If you believe you are unworthy, not good enough, unlovable, or flawed in some way, and also believe that being slim and attractive would make you more valuable, sabotaging your weight loss efforts and keeping you fat is a great way for your subconscious to affirm these negative beliefs to you. Inversely, you can't believe that you are worthwhile, lovable, more than good enough, and deserve the best life has to offer and continue to be significantly overweight and in poor health if you believe that being slim and healthy correlates—at any level—to desirability, value, or worth.

The purpose of this book is not to debate the morality of linking value to physical attractiveness, or physical attractiveness to how much you weigh. I think most of us can agree in a perfect world we would all be valued and loved based on who we are and not what we look like. Unfortunately that isn't the world we live in. The idea that physical attractiveness in some way creates value, and that being overweight diminishes physical attractiveness, is a cultural level belief that permeates our society. Therefore, no matter what we want to believe, it's almost impossible that these judgments are not in some way a part of us subconsciously even if we consciously choose to reject them.

Our subconscious will work with whatever material we give it to prove what we believe about ourselves to be true. In a culture where physical attractiveness and slim bodies are prized and correlate in any way to a person being seen as more valuable or lovable, your subconscious will often act on beliefs related to your own lack of self-worth or value by making you overweight. However, if we were to go back several hundred years we would find an era where carrying extra body fat was seen as very attractive in women and a sign of affluence with men. In that era and in that culture, your subconscious wouldn't use obesity to prove to you that any negative beliefs about yourself were true because there weren't the same inferences between body fat and unattractiveness that you find in our culture.

The reverse side of this is to think that being slim will make you happy. That's another false belief that we will dismantle on our journey together. When done with the program, you may or may not have the body that you presently think will make you happy, but you will have the body that the happiness you find builds. I promise that will be far better than what you are imagining now.

Do I believe you can be truly happy, have cleared your negative beliefs about yourself, healed your emotional wounds, and reprogram your subconscious for success in life and still be significantly overweight? It's possible, but in our society not likely. I would also say that those select few that manage to find happiness while being overweight aren't the ones blogging and talking about it, they're busy living their lives and being happy, while the latter group is perhaps protesting too much while in denial.

If you are one of the few that are significantly overweight and are happy with it, then this book isn't for you. If, however, you've picked up this book for any reason, regardless of what you tell yourself, I would propose that you may not be as happy being overweight as you think. The litmus test for this is your own emotional reactions to what I've written so far. If you feel offended, angry, or have any type of strong emotional reaction, it's an indication that we've touched upon some unhealed emotional wounds that are intertwined with your body and your weight. In this book I'm going to expose you to concepts that are going to create an emotional reaction. That means that sometimes you may not like what I have to say very much and possibly dislike me by association. That's ok, I like me, and when we are done together "you" liking "you" in a way that allows you to lose weight and keep it off is all that matters to me. As I've already said, you have to feel it to heal it. We have work to do together. Let's get started.

HOW TO USE THIS BOOK

This book combines the most powerful methods and techniques available in the world today to create lasting weight loss from the inside out. My experience over years of creating long-term and lifelong weight loss success with my clients is based on the study and integration of multiple disciplines. As a Certified Personal Trainer and Medical Exercise Specialist, I found that I could hold people's hands long enough to get them to their goal, and because they did not change the underlying emotional issues, they always regained the weight. There was definitely something missing.

As I added additional training and credentials, I found that Clinical Hypnotherapy, Cognitive Behavioral Coaching, Neuro-Linguistic Programming, and EFT Therapies all held part of the answer to creating long-term success—but all were missing something. It was only when I combined and synthesized these modalities into a comprehensive approach that addressed all the areas that cause people to be overweight that my clients began achieving the goals that they had spent a lifetime dreaming of. They didn't just lose weight, but also changed the way they felt about themselves, food, and their bodies in a way that allowed them to easily keep it off.

One of the reasons a multi-disciplined approach is so effective is because not everyone benefits equally from the same methods. In this book you will find that some of the information, techniques, and neural technologies seem as if they were made just for you, while others work well but do not seem to have the same fit. That is why this book is full of resources and self-diagnostic criteria. It is to allow you to find and understand what works best for you, and then to have more than enough of those specific resources to make the changes in your weight, your body, and your mind that you desire.

The book also features several testimonials from past clients to help you relate and better understand and apply the material. All names have been changed to protect these clients' identities and maintain client confidentiality.

As you go through the book, workbook, video tutorials, and audio sessions, it is important to try all of the processes and exercises. You will find that some exercises that do not seem ideal for you now will be perfect for you later as you grow and evolve through the *Fat to Fearless*® program. It is important to understand that you can't create subconscious change academically or intellectually. Change is created through feeling and emotion, and to get the results you want, you must do the exercises and go through the process.

At the end of each significant section and chapter you will find a summary that consists of the following three components:

Key Points

In this area I will summarize the preceding section or chapter into very easily understandable points that are important for you to take away from your reading.

What This Has To Do With Weight Loss

Here, I will specifically explain what the material you just read and the concepts you just learned have to do with losing weight and keeping it off. Some of the concepts in *Fat to Fearless*® allow you to heal deep emotional wounds that affect many areas of your life. This is where I will specifically focus on the previous learnings' application to weight loss.

You Are Ready To Move To The Next Chapter When . . .

It's important to not go through the material too quickly. This is a process and an experience; the pace at which you go through it is to be determined by how quickly you experience change, not how quickly you can read. In this section I will give you criteria for helping you assess when you're ready to move on to the next chapter or section of the program.

If you only have the book, you are missing significant parts of the program. *Fat to Fearless®* is a set of understandings, principles, and techniques that are built upon the foundation of the recorded Clinical Hypnotherapy sessions and interactive video instructional sessions that, along with the Success Guide and Workbook, comprise the entire system. Certainly, the book will have value on its own, but if you are serious about creating lasting change in both your body and your mind, I highly encourage you to invest in yourself by getting the entire program at www.fattofearless.com.

Do Not try to accomplish the *Fat to Fearless®* program by just reading the chapter summaries!

Writing a book and creating a system like *Fat to Fearless®* requires putting steps and what you learn into a linear process. However, many of the processes actually occur simultaneously in live therapy. Because of this, you will not only find that you make significant leaps forward as you go through each module and section in order, but that once you've completed the entire program and combine all of the skills learned so that you can apply them simultaneously, you will then make additional progress even faster. Many people find great value in repeating the *Fat to Fearless®* program, finding that each time they learn something new about themselves and how to apply that knowledge, they improve their lives in areas beyond weight loss.

I have put a great deal of information into this book. I could easily have elaborated on many of the understandings in *Fat to Fearless®* and created three separate books. Instead, I decided to include as much as possible in this one book and program. The advantage to that is that you have a resource that will guide you through any emotional or subconscious difficulty you may have in losing weight if you take the time to fully go through the program. The downside of so much information is that you may feel overwhelmed if you don't allow yourself the time, as well as the attention needed, to fully go through the book, workbook, and videos. *Don't be in a rush.* Take your time and allow yourself to fully experience each step of the journey as you learn new skills and adapt to different ways of thinking and feeling about your body. Throughout the program, the chapter summaries as well as the video tutorials will simplify everything into easy-to-understand actions and principles.

I also highly recommend that you download my free Getting Started video at www.asherfoxweightloss.com/gettingstarted before you begin the program.

FREE UPDATES, RESOURCES, AND GIFTS

*F*at *to Fearless*® is not just a book, methodology, or program; it is a mindset and a community. I have created several resources to not only help you connect, support, and be supported by others just like you, but to also help me share bonus content, answer your questions, and interact with you personally. I highly encourage you to maximize your weight loss success by taking advantage of these resources and joining the following communities:

Facebook

On our Facebook fan page you can connect with others just like you. I also share testimonial videos and inspirational stories from participants, as well as tips and best practices for going through the program. Please "like us" on Facebook to take advantage of these great resources.

www.facebook.com/asherfoxweightloss

Private Social Media Community

Asherfoxweightloss.org is my free, private *Fat to Fearless*® social media community where I personally answer your questions, give away newly developed tools and resources, as well as provide free updates to the program. Here you can find accountability and support partners and join small groups focused specifically on the areas of the *Fat to Fearless*® program that you are the most interested in. You can even get advice and support from those who have already achieved their weight loss goals using *Fat to Fearless*®.

Also, you can visit the community resource center and find several exclusive free discounts for community members on products, programs, and services offered by major companies and brands that can support you on your weight loss journey.

www.asherfoxweightloss.org

Twitter

Twitter is our way of keeping you motivated and on track throughout the day while you are going from *Fat to Fearless*®. Follow us on Twitter, where I provide additional Twitter-only bonus downloads as well as those daily reminders that will keep you focused on your goal in a healthy and fun way.

www.twitter.com/asherfox

The Asher Fox Show

Be sure to join me on my weekly call-in radio show where each week I discuss weight loss with a guest expert, along with a variety of other topics ranging from relationship and dating issues to healing the heart and many other topics relevant to living your best possible life. Information about the Asher Fox Show, including days, times, and topics can be found at the website below:

www.theasherfoxshow.com

OTHER PROGRAMS

*F*at to Fearless® is not a diet, nutrition, or exercise program, yet it can be combined with many of these with great results. *Fat to Fearless*® addresses the root emotional and psychological causes of why people commonly fail to stick with healthy eating and exercise long enough to lose weight, and commonly gain back what they do lose through self-sabotaging behavior.

All of our outcomes, in all areas of our lives, including our bodies and our weight, begin in the mind and heart. This program addresses those root causes in a powerfully transformative way. However, to lose weight and be healthy still requires eating well and getting appropriate activity. For this reason, any nutrition or fitness program that is physically healthy for you can be an excellent companion on your *Fat to Fearless*® journey.

To receive a list of weight loss plans and fitness programs we endorse, as well as discounts to many of these, be sure to join our free community at www.fattofearless.org.

THE *FAT TO FEARLESS*® FOUNDATION

If you've invested in this book, then you are either very aware that the root cause of your inability to lose weight lies more in your head and your heart (emotions) than in your body, or at the very least you are looking for answers that you've yet to find about why you haven't been able to achieve permanent weight loss. If you're like most of the clients I've had over almost 20 years of specializing in mind/body transformation, it's taken a lot of failed attempts at traditional diets and exercise programs to bring you to the point where you are ready to look deeper within yourself to find these answers.

The foundation of the *Fat to Fearless*® program is based on two proven presuppositions that you must accept to create permanent weight loss success. They are:

1. Your subconscious Core Beliefs are acted upon as blueprints that your subconscious uses to construct your life. This includes your body and your ability to lose weight and keep it off.

2. Traditional diet/exercise attempts based on conscious willpower to lose weight don't work because of The Symptom Cycle. The Symptom Cycle states that the way you feel about a symptom creates behaviors based on those emotions that ultimately are the cause of the original symptoms. For our purposes, symptoms can be

defined as the self-sabotaging behaviors that have kept you from losing weight and keeping it off.

While it isn't necessary that you accept both of these presuppositions as true at this point, as the program itself will prove them to you, it is essential that you at least be open to the concepts. Let's briefly look at each principal now:

Core Beliefs Act as Blueprints for Your Life

I've already briefly touched on this concept and it will be greatly elaborated on throughout the book, but it's an important principle to understand at the beginning. Core beliefs are things that we believe about ourselves, the world around us, and the very nature of life at a subconscious level. These beliefs, often formed in childhood, act as an "operating system" for our lives. Some of these beliefs we are aware of, but since they exist at the subconscious level, many of them we are not.

Core beliefs have so much influence in our lives because one of the primary functions of the subconscious mind is to prove itself right. The idea being that if we constantly changed and tested what we believe at a fundamental level, we could put ourselves in danger. This is a survival mechanism that developed early in our evolution. A good way of illustrating this is to think about when people used to believe the world was flat.

The belief that the world was flat was a core societal belief that was almost universally shared, and part of this belief was that if you sailed too far out you could actually fall off the end of the world. Multiple experiments and first-hand experiences of the day seemed to confirm this as a reality despite us now knowing the world is round. The reason that it took so long for man to find out the truth about our planet's shape was that the subconscious of everyone that held this belief was heavily invested in making sure that, no matter what "reality" was, no one came to any conclusion that would cause them to do something so foolish as possibly risk falling off the edge of the known world.

The subconscious mind is interested in our survival based on what has "worked" for us in the past. No one was going to die from believing the world was flat, but there was a chance you could end your life by testing some crazy new theory about a round world. You can see how a subconscious mechanism that kept us acting in line with what had worked for us so far and avoided us trying on every new belief that came along was an evolutionary advantage.

Once our subconscious accepts something as a known fact it obscures our ability to see beyond that belief because it interprets our core beliefs as "rules to live by." Subsequently, using a variety of mechanisms you're going to learn about in this book, it ensures we never form a different conclusion because it "stacks the deck" against us by driving us to behaviors that seem to prove these beliefs are true. This is why all of the evidence during that time in history was interpreted as confirming a flat world. Their subconscious minds ensured they saw things that way.

While this may have been a useful survival mechanism at some point in our early evolution, as we evolved and became more complex in our thinking and our ability to feel emotions, this rule designed to always ensure we lived out what we believed began to be applied to what we thought about ourselves and our self-worth.

If you had experiences early in life that caused you to form the beliefs that you were unlovable, not good enough, a failure, or deficient in any way, your subconscious mind takes these beliefs and uses them to construct the boundaries of your world. After all, believing you're not good enough, or unattractive, or second best has gotten you this far in life so why risk changing it?

The subconscious mind deals in what is "known," which means it deals in what it has previously interpreted to be true. If living with these beliefs has allowed you to survive so far, changing these beliefs creates the one thing that the subconscious always interprets as dangerous—the unknown.

In a desire to keep you "safe," your subconscious causes you to interpret experiences in such a way, while also driving you to behaviors, that seems to reaffirm these beliefs to you. If you have the belief that you are "less than" in any way, and you also believe that being overweight makes you less valuable or less attractive as a person, then you've given your subconscious mind the perfect way to prove your negative core beliefs about yourself true. As long as it ensures you stay overweight, you will always believe you are "less than," which, since it's kept you alive so far, will ensure you stay within the boundaries that the subconscious mind considers to be safe for you.

The challenge comes when our conscious mind determines it wants something different and new from what the subconscious mind considers to be proven and safe. If you've struggled with significant lifelong weight issues, this conflict between your conscious and your subconscious mind is at the heart of that struggle.

You are reading this book because you consciously want to lose weight and end your lifelong struggle with excess pounds. Our job together is going to be to change the beliefs that you now have about yourself in a way that changes the boundaries of your life to encompass a new world, one in which your subconscious accepts and believes it would be best for you to be thinner. Once this happens, you will be amazed at the change in both your body and in how you feel about yourself.

Let's now look at the second presupposition.

The Symptom Cycle

It's important to understand in more detail why focusing on losing weight through more "direct" fitness and nutrition approaches alone typically doesn't work if you're someone who has suffered from weight issues most of their life.

I'll begin by explaining what I mean when I say "someone who has suffered from weight issues most of their life." Obviously, there are a lot of people who are trying to lose weight that haven't been overweight for a significant period of time. Many of these people have gained weight as a result of age (unless we are taking steps to prevent it, our metabolism slows every year starting in our mid-20s) or a change in lifestyle (retirement or a new desk job). For these people, there aren't necessarily deep subconscious reasons that have caused them to gain weight.

One of the things that you will learn is that what's in our subconscious tends to not change on its own. When an inability to lose weight is rooted in the subconscious, as is the case with emotional eating, it tends to be a lifelong problem. Another indicator that a weight issue has its origins in our subconscious is how extreme the weight problem is.

Someone who just needs to lose 5 or 10 pounds is typically dealing with issues around lifestyle, body type, aging, and other factors. However, if you've struggled with 20 or more pounds most of your life it's a sure bet that part of the problem lies in emotional eating. As you will most definitely learn, emotional eating is rooted in the subconscious.

For those people who only have a small amount of weight to lose, and it hasn't been a lifelong issue, it can usually be addressed through traditional weight loss and exercise programs. Often, because these individuals are used to being able to maintain their weight with the lifestyle they had before their metabolism slowed with age or their lifestyle became more sedentary, they do need to increase their willpower as it relates to food and exercise. For those individuals I recommend my book and program Weight Loss Willpower and Movement Motivation™. However, if you have a significant amount of weight to lose and suffer from emotional eating, those emotions and subconscious programming will always beat conscious "willpower." Therefore, the only long-term solution is to reprogram the subconscious and heal the mind so that you no longer turn to food for comfort.

If this describes you, the reason that focusing exclusively on the direct approach to weight loss (dieting and exercise, etc.) never works long term is because of what's called the Symptom Cycle. The Symptom Cycle says that the way we feel about a symptom is the cause of the symptom. Let me show you how this pertains to weight loss.

Let's begin by defining the word symptom. According to Webster's dictionary:

Symptom: a change in the body or mind which indicates that a disease is present, a change which shows that something bad exists, a sign of something bad.

When I talk about the symptom, I'm talking about being overweight and/or the behaviors that make you overweight. When treating a problem, you always try to treat the source of the problem and not the actual symptom. When you go to the doctor for an infection, he doesn't just give you medication to make you feel better but gives you medication to try to eliminate the infection altogether. So now that we know that the symptom is being overweight, let's put that into the context of the Symptom Cycle.

As I explained, the Symptom Cycle says that the way that we feel about the symptom is the cause of the symptom. In other words, the way that we feel about being overweight is the cause of being overweight. Let's do an exercise to illustrate the concept.

EXERCISE: THE SYMPTOM CYCLE

Step 1
Close your eyes and find a memory of the last time you were feeling really overweight. Maybe it was a time that you had just gotten out of the shower and caught a glimpse of yourself in the mirror, or perhaps when you were trying to put on clothes that didn't fit, or possibly even a time when someone said something negative about your body. Make this memory as real as you can in your mind's eye.

Now, feeling these emotions, open your eyes and write down what word you call yourself when you feel the worst about your body. This isn't a time to censor yourself but a time to be completely honest. For some the word is "fat," for others it's more vague and might be "disgusting," or perhaps something unique to you.

When you have that word, put it into the following sentence and complete the sentence with your first reaction without giving it any thought first or editing your response:

Being *(insert your word)* makes me feel so _____.

Now write that word down in the space provided in your Success Guide and Workbook. Next, I want you to do the exact same thing again, filling in the blank with a different word. Continue doing this until you start repeating the same words.

When you're done, you should have filled in the blanks with approximately 5 to 10 words that describe how you feel about being overweight. Some common examples are: sad, angry, overwhelmed, ugly, helpless, guilty, etc.

If you now go back to the Symptom Cycle you will see that you have a list of emotions that define "how you feel about the symptom."

Step 2

Now close your eyes again and this time go back to the last time you ate for emotional reasons. Perhaps you indulged in foods that you knew would set you back or maybe you just ate more than you should have.

Once you are in that memory, make a list of everything you were feeling at the time. Specifically, what emotions you were trying to soothe through food. Perhaps at the time you didn't think of it in that way, but looking at it now in hindsight, list those emotions in the appropriate blanks in your Success Guide and Workbook.

You now have a list of the emotions that are the cause of the symptom "overeating." Overeating is of course also the cause of being overweight. For the purposes of this exercise we will consider the two synonymous.

Step 3

Compare the two lists. You will notice that, if not identical, the lists are very similar. In other words, the way you *feel about being overweight* is the same set of emotions that cause you to engage in the behaviors that *cause you to be overweight.*

This exercise gives you an understanding of how the Symptom Cycle applies to body transformation. You're overeating to try to feel better about how you feel about yourself, which is in part because of how you feel about your body. You can now begin to understand why only focusing on the symptom will never yield long-term results.

When you only focus on the symptom, being overweight, you can never lose weight fast enough to reach your goal before the bad feelings you have about your body cause you to engage in emotional eating and sabotage your progress. When you add to that other psychological mechanisms that cause us to engage in all or nothing behavior, making what could be only momentary dietary slips turn into days of unhealthy eating, it becomes even easier to see why you must deal not just with the symptoms, but with the underlying causes as well.

As you go through the *Fat to Fearless*® program you are going to transform the underlying negative emotions that cause you to overeat and eat the wrong foods for reasons other than hunger into healthier emotions that support you in losing weight. You're also going to discover that you don't feel bad because you are overweight but have been overweight because you felt bad about yourself. Through this journey into your subconscious mind you're probably going to also discover that you felt this way at a very young age before you even became overweight and that ultimately your subconscious acted on these feelings to create the body you now have. You're going to finally learn which came first, the chicken or the egg, and the answer might surprise you.

Body, Mind, and Soul Goals

It is important to begin a journey with an understanding of the destination, especially when that destination seems to be a place you have tried to reach before but is actually quite different. This journey is going to require a whole new map.

It is common when beginning a weight loss program, diet, or fitness plan, to set goals such as reaching a particular weight, losing a certain number of pounds per week, or fitting into a certain size of clothing. Few people, however, set goals for how they want to feel or how they want their life to change on an emotional level. We make assumptions about how we will feel, thinking it will happen automatically, when the scale finally reveals that magic number.

Did you know that over 70% of lottery winners are broke again within 5 years? The reason is that they too made assumptions about how their lives would change if they had money. However, they didn't make the changes inside that allowed them to believe they deserved the wealth. When you change your "outside" without changing your "inside," you will subconsciously sabotage yourself to ensure that your life circumstances match your internal beliefs. The lottery winner will suddenly find themselves broke again, and the dieter will regain their weight.

This is what happens with weight loss if you do not do the deep inner work to change your subconscious beliefs to match the body you want. At best you reach your weight loss goals for only a short period of time before, just like the lottery winners going broke, you regain the weight.

It seems like the deeper the issue or problem, the more we search for answers on the surface. Nowhere is this more true than when we try to alleviate the hurt inside by dropping pounds on the outside. Many people go through life believing that their self-worth can be measured by the number on a scale. Most people will never admit how much they view their value through "fat-colored glasses" in a way that diminishes, in almost every area, their experience of life.

Unfortunately, if you have suffered from chronic weight issues for most of your life, healing your hurts cannot be accomplished without facing and feeling painful emotions within yourself. This is not a book about learning to love yourself in spite of being overweight, but about realizing that learning to love yourself is absolutely essential to losing weight and keeping it off forever.

As you will soon learn, changing only your body does not create lasting subconscious change. Without changing the subconscious parts of yourself that force you to self-sabotage, you will eventually regain whatever weight you lose. On this particular journey, you are headed in two places that at first seem fundamentally different but are really just mirror images of each other. The destination you seek is one that is both inside of you and outside of you, yet are the same. Put simply, the body you seek on the outside will be a mirror reflection of the high self-esteem and self-love you develop on the inside by going through the *Fat to Fearless*® process.

It is important to define your internal and external goals because it is possible to lose weight in the short term without learning to love or value yourself, which is why the pounds always come back. When you evaluate your progress not only on how your body changes, but also how you change mentally and emotionally, you are able to keep weight off for a lifetime.

Every week, just as you check the scale to see how much weight you lose, check with yourself to see what is going on inside. The *Fat to Fearless*® program gives you the tools to do this. When you determine you are off course, whether for your weight loss goals or your deeper goals of self-love and self-esteem, you will have the tools to get back on course and start making progress again.

While losing weight and keeping it off will definitely bring many improvements to your life, your life will not automatically transform into everything you want because of it. If your self-esteem is based on how you look instead of who you are, self-loathing, negative judgments, and bad feelings will never be more than a few cupcakes behind.

Decide how you want to feel about yourself, and make a plan to get there. When you use techniques that are proven to work, and then use your internal change as the motivation to transform your body, you will find you keep your weight off because you transformed yourself from the inside out.

EXERCISE: BODY, MIND, AND SOUL GOALS

Now is the time to set your goals. If you have the *Fat to Fearless*® Success Guide and Workbook, go to the appropriate exercise and follow the steps. If you do no have the workbook, answer the following on a sheet of paper:

1. How am I going to evaluate my weight loss progress? A goal weight? How my clothes fit? Energy level?

2. Set your goals using whatever criteria is best for you.

3. Why are these particular goals important to me?

4. How do I want to feel about myself: While I am in the process of losing weight? After I reach my goal weight?

5. Regardless of how my body looks, if I could magically feel that way about myself now, how would my life change even if my body stayed the same? At first you might say, "I couldn't feel that way if my body did not change," but pretend you could and did. Your imagination is going to be a powerful ally on this journey.

6. How do I want my life to be different once I reach my goal weight?

7. List 5 things you will do, be, or have once you reach your goal weight. These are 5 things that are very motivating to you.

Note on Setting a Goal Weight

In the *Fat to Fearless*® Success Guide and Workbook, I review physical guidelines for healthy weight loss. If you do not have the workbook, just know that I recommend you lose no more than 1 to 2 pounds per week.

Plotting Your Course

Unlike other programs that focus on the physical aspects of diet and nutrition, this book and the *Fat to Fearless*® program do not address the symptoms (what and how you eat, or specific exercise programs), but instead go straight to the root causes, which are your beliefs, your emotions and the behaviors they cause. Going from being fat and feeling helpless to having the body you want and living life fearlessly will lead you through the following terrain:

Your Mind: An Owner's Manual

First, you are going to get a brief tutorial on how everyone's mind works, specifically your conscious mind, subconscious mind, and how they interact, as well as what rules those interactions follow.

Your Beliefs and Your Body

You are going to learn about your core beliefs, those you are aware and unaware of, and the role they play in subconsciously driving your behavior and creating your body. You'll understand how these beliefs are formed and learn about all of the subconscious mechanism's that have previously kept you from changing these beliefs to ones that support you in reaching your goals. You'll also learn how to bypass these previously sabotaging mechanisms to allow you to create the deep inner changes you seek.

New Body Beliefs

Here, you are going to actually begin the process of changing your uncovered core beliefs into ones that support you in reaching your body transformation goals. You will learn how to take the previously learned ways that your subconscious works against you and get them to work for you instead. Through a proven step-by-step process, you will identify the beliefs you do not want, change them into the ones that you do want, and reprogram your subconscious mind for weight loss success.

Eating and Your Emotions

Your emotions drive your behaviors. If you want to change what you do and the results you get, you must change how you feel inside. You will learn how to get in touch with your deep emotional self and transform the negative emotions that have driven you to eat mindlessly into positive ones that motivate you to live life fully without using food as a crutch to feel better.

Living Fearlessly

You have managed to accomplish a lot in other areas of your life despite obstacles and difficulty, so why has losing weight been such a challenge? As you pass through this part of the program, you will come to understand hidden motivations based on unconcious fears that cause your subconscious to self-sabotage your success because it actually believes you are better off staying overweight. Changing this will make weight loss easier than it's ever been before.

As you move through each of these areas, you will find answers to the questions about why you have never been able to lose weight and keep it off. You will learn how to apply these answers to create lasting transformation. Finally, you will arrive at your destination, not only with the body you want, but with lasting positive emotions and high self-esteem.

Through this interdependent relationship between your physical body and your emotional self, you will create a lasting inner/outer balance that will reinforce, regulate, and maintain your weight and your positive feelings for a lifetime.

By the end of our time together, you will achieve your goals with your body, transform your emotions and your mind, and set your soul free to live fearlessly. You will have reached your Body-Mind-Soul goals.

Let's get to work!

PART II

YOUR MIND:
AN OWNER'S MANUAL

CHAPTER 1

UNDERSTANDING YOUR SUBCONSCIOUS

Our journey into changing your behavior, like the behaviors that lead to being overweight, begins with understanding the subconscious mind. But what exactly is the subconscious mind, how do we know we have one, and what is the difference between our conscious and subconscious?

The conscious mind is the part of our mind that we are aware of: our daily thoughts, the memories we are aware of, and our thinking and reasoning. For most people, it is who they believe they are.

The subconscious mind is the part of us responsible for all mental activities that take place below conscious awareness. This includes everything we consciously do not acknowledge: memories that are too distant or traumatic to recall, information that comes in through our senses that is determined to not be important, our core beliefs, as well as the origins of our emotional reactions. Our subconscious minds also control our autonomic nervous system which is responsible for the bodily functions that work without our actively thinking about them (breathing, digestion, metabolism, etc.).

Any of our mental or psychic functions that we are not aware of are controlled by the subconscious or unconscious mind (for our purposes the terms subconscious and unconscious are interchangeable). Opinions about how and why the subconscious exists and is formed range from our psychological need to not deal with certain experiences to the biological understanding of how our brains developed in phases during different stages of evolution. But the origin of our subconscious is something we will leave to scientists, researchers, and philosophers. We want to understand how the subconscious keeps us overweight and how to change that.

One of the first questions my clients ask is, "Which is more powerful, the conscious or the subconscious mind?" The following list not only answers that question, but helps you understand why your subconscious is important in going from *Fat to Fearless*®.

The subconscious mind processes information at a staggering rate. The processing power of the subconscious is staggering when compared to the conscious mind. According to Dr. Bruce Lipton in his book, *The Biology of Belief*, the conscious mind can only process 40 bits of information per second while the subconscious mind can process 20,000 bits of information per second. This means the subconscious mind is 500 times faster than the conscious mind. While these numbers differ depending upon the studies cited, the differences are only slight. All research concurs that the subconscious has an exponentially greater processing capacity than the conscious mind.

The subconscious mind is like a massive hard drive. The subconscious stores every experience you have ever had since your brain was able to record experiences, and it retains all of this information for a lifetime. Even though your conscious mind does not remember everything, all of your memories are stored safely away in your subconscious. This includes memories you may not be able to recall but still actively influence your life.

Emotions are generated from the subconscious. Since emotion is always a more powerful motivating force than reason and logic, this is another way that the subconscious trumps the conscious mind in influencing our behavior. While we can influence how we feel by using our conscious mind, the change in emotion is usually because of how the subconscious is responding to that conscious effort.

The subconscious controls the autonomic nervous system and influences all functions of the body. Even cell growth and DNA are influenced by our subconscious and the emotional states that arise within it. With the ability to change hormone levels, metabolic rate, and even the manifestation of disease and sickness, the subconscious can take your body hostage anytime it wants.

Our lack of knowing what is in the subconscious gives it power. The term "subconscious" means unconscious. Not the type of unconsciousness you experience when you are sleeping, but not having conscious awareness. Since you do not consciously know about what it's doing, the subconscious is often free to do what it does in the shadows, even if it's in direct contradiction to what you consciously want. Without full awareness of what is actually going on, your conscious mind loses much of its ability to interfere with the subconscious' agenda. If you have been struggling to lose weight your entire life and have never kept it off, it is likely that your subconscious has an agenda and a reason to keep you overweight that hasn't been shared with your conscious mind.

The subconscious mind never sleeps. While your conscious mind checks out for eight hours or so a day, the subconscious mind is functioning every second of every minute of every day of your life. If your conscious and subconscious mind are in conflict and want separate things, your subconscious mind has an extra eight hours a day to achieve its goals while your conscious mind has gone off to slumber. It is also working with 500 times more processing power! Now you know why the subconscious is always the winner.

The subconscious mind is the home of our core beliefs. Later you will learn in more detail how core beliefs are formed and stored in the subconscious, but for now know that everything you believe about yourself and the world around you at the deepest level is in the subconscious mind. Some of these beliefs you are consciously aware of while others you are not. For example, if you have core beliefs that you are a fat person, do not deserve to be happy, or are deficient in any way, these beliefs are stored in the subconscious. Soon you will understand what the subconscious does with these beliefs and how that impacts your success in all areas of life, including weight loss.

The subconscious mind is the source of all of our creativity. This is because creativity is the process of taking different, often unrelated concepts and ideas, and recombining pieces of them to form new ideas. All those old concepts and ideas are stored in your subconscious. Edison would often solve his challenges related to new inventions by taking short naps and asking his subconscious to solve the problems for him. Many times he awoke with the perfect creative solution. Part of being able to reinvent yourself, including reinventing your body, is finding new, creative ways to look at food, yourself, and life. Synthesizing creative ideas and solutions is one of the subconscious mind's most important functions.

The subconscious mind filters information to our conscious mind based on our unconscious beliefs. You will learn more about the brain's Reticular Activating System (R.A.S.), which determines what we consciously become aware of, and how it is influenced by the subconscious. We tend to notice things that support maintaining our subconscious core beliefs. In other words, if we believe we can or cannot do anything, our subconscious mind influences all the millions of bits of information that come in every second to ensure that the 40 bits of information we become conscious of support us in that belief. Whether we believe the glass is half-empty or half-full, our subconscious mind proves us right by providing only the evidence that supports what we believe. Every day that we do not become conscious of what our subconscious is doing and take active steps to ensure our subconscious is working toward our conscious goals, we create and live a self-fulfilling prophecy of our deepest beliefs, which unfortunately are sometimes in direct opposition to what we say or think we want for our lives.

The subconscious mind directs our energy and resources. Both directly through control of the autonomic nervous system and indirectly through our emotions, how much energy we have for almost every activity is strongly influenced by what is going on in our subconscious. For those who do not enjoy exercise or feel tired all day, it's easy to see how important this aspect of the subconscious mind is to long-term lifestyle change.

The subconscious mind carries out our habitual conduct. Nothing determines the direction of our life more than our habits. Habits are usually unconscious patterns of behavior that happen almost automatically with little to no effort. Habits are essential for our basic functioning. Think of how little we would get done if we had to stop and consciously think about all of our behaviors throughout the day. Habits allow us to be efficient by putting much of our daily tasks on autopilot.

While habits can be very positive, they can also work against us because some habits developed out of our unhealthy core beliefs (using food to "feel better" for instance). To go from *Fat to Fearless®*, which by definition means keeping the weight off, requires creating new habits in place of the old ones that allow you to put your weight maintenance on auto pilot.

The subconscious always seeks to make itself right. Once a core belief has been accepted by the subconscious mind, it uses the previously mentioned filtering system and other mechanisms to prove to your conscious mind that those beliefs are true. We are living lives created by our subconscious core beliefs that we may not be aware of. When we become aware of those beliefs and replace the ones we do not want with ones that serve us, our subconscious then begins to recreate our experience of life based on our new beliefs.

One of my favorite analogies for the subconscious mind is that of a ship and its captain. The conscious mind is like the captain who makes decisions and gives orders about where to direct the ship (in this metaphor, the ship is your life). Everyone else on the ship—the engineers, the navigator, the communications officer, the cook, and the men in the boiler room shoveling coal into the steam engines—are your subconscious mind.

While the captain can give orders all day long, the ship only moves in the direction he wants when the rest of the crew follows his orders. If he says to go south, but the navigator directs the ship north instead, or the crew in the engine room decides they don't want to go anywhere and then shut down the engines, the captain's orders mean nothing.

The ship only functions like it is supposed to when the captain and crew work together, just like your life only goes the way you truly want it to when your conscious and subconscious mind are aligned toward the same goals.

While you will learn much more about the subconscious mind on your *Fat to Fearless*® journey, these basic understandings of why and how the subconscious mind truly dominates your life, usually in ways you are not even aware, should be eye opening.

Next you are going to learn about the Weight Loss Laws of the Mind. If you understand how the subconscious works together with the Weight Loss Laws of the Mind, you will understand why you have found it difficult to permanently lose weight. You will also learn the reasons behind not reaching many of your other goals in life.

SUMMARY

Key Points

- The conscious mind is the part of the mind we are aware of. It's responsible for our reasoning, analytical thinking, and goal setting. It's with our conscious mind that we make the decision that we want to lose weight and plan how we are going to go about it.

- The subconscious mind is the part of our mind we are *not* aware of. It houses all of our memories from the time our brains were developed enough to actually store information. Our core beliefs, habits, compulsions, and self-sabotaging behavior originates from our subconscious mind. If we consciously say we want to lose weight and keep it off but have never reached that goal, it is most likely that what's in our subconscious is in conflict with that goal.

- The term "subconscious mind" is interchangeable with the term "unconscious mind."

- By definition, when something is in the subconscious we are unconscious of it; we are unaware of it. For this reason, many people refuse to believe their subconscious is responsible for their weight loss difficulties because they consciously don't intend to self-sabotage.

- The conscious mind is responsible for approximately 8% to 12% of our mental functioning, as compared to the 88% to 92% of the subconscious mind. In addition, the subconscious has 500 times more processing power than the conscious mind.

- The nature of the subconscious mind is that we are often unaware of our hidden beliefs and what the subconscious believes is best for us.

- What we consciously want for our lives is often different from what we subconsciously believe is best, based on hidden beliefs from childhood that we are unaware of.

- When what we consciously want is in conflict with what the subconscious wants—the subconscious always wins.

- Changing any lifelong behaviors, such as behaviors that lead to being overweight, requires change at the subconscious level if it's going to last.

What This Has To Do With Weight Loss

Almost all of our behavior is either driven or influenced by the subconscious mind. Examples of subconsciously driven behaviors are emotional eating, mindless eating, and self-sabotage (especially regaining lost weight). Through the *Fat to Fearless*® program you will begin to change your subconscious so it supports you in reaching your goals. Part of that process is learning how your subconscious mind works.

You Are Ready To Move To The Next Chapter When . . .

- You have a solid understanding of how much more powerful the subconscious is than the conscious mind and why creating permanent change in an area of your life that you've struggled with, such as weight loss, requires subconscious change.

- You have watched the tutorial video for this chapter and are following the included instructions to actively use your Hypnotherapy Audio Sessions (if you have the full *Fat to Fearless*® program).

- You are listening to your Hypnotherapy Audio Sessions according to their included instructions (if you have the full *Fat to Fearless*® program).

CHAPTER 2

WEIGHT LOSS LAWS OF THE MIND

The Laws of the Mind are like a user's manual for the subconscious. For our purposes, I have renamed them the Weight Loss Laws of the Mind because we are going to specifically be dealing with how they apply to weight loss even though they can also be applied to any area of your life. When you understand these laws, you can stop working against your subconscious and begin enlisting its help to reach all of your goals, including losing weight. If the subconscious mind were a lock, then the Weight Loss Laws of the Mind would be the key. These laws will unlock your subconscious to give you secret access to the tools you need to transform your body and your life. You will learn about them in this chapter and later in the program you will begin actively applying this knowledge.

As you read through the Weight Loss Laws of the Mind, ask yourself how they might give insight into the behaviors that have kept you from achieving long-term success either in weight loss or any other area. If you have the *Fat to Fearless*® Success Guide and Workbook, be sure to do this chapter's exercise where you can list your insights on how each law has either worked for you or against you. If you don't have the full program with the workbook and videos, I would encourage you to invest in yourself by downloading it from:

www.fattofearless.com

Otherwise, complete the exercise on your own paper by writing down any awareness that comes to mind on how you can see these laws having worked in your own life. At this point in the program, you may not have a lot of insight into this yet, but do the exercise anyway. Later, when it all starts to come together, you can come back and fill your answers in more.

1. **The Law of Reverse Effect**

   The Law of Reverse Effect tells us that the greater the conscious effort, the less the subconscious mind responds. You've probably had the experience of trying to remember something, perhaps a name or telephone number, and the harder you try to remember, the less you are able to. But as soon as you stop trying and put your mind on something else, the answer quickly pops into your head. This is the Law of Reverse Effect at work.

   Another example is when you try to force yourself to exercise or not eat that last cupcake. The more you try, the harder it becomes, until eventually you give in. This law works based on what you are focusing on. When you are trying to remember the number, your focus is on the fact that you can't remember it. Whenever you are trying to resist food, your focus is on the desire for it. The subconscious responds to what you focus on.

   This law, in part, explains why you have had so much difficulty sticking to your program. Since you know that "not trying" to resist temptation also didn't work, it is important to understand this is only one part of the puzzle. By the time you complete the *Fat to Fearless®* program, you will have a complete understanding of the tools you need to change self-defeating behaviors and work with, not against, your subconscious mind.

2. The Law of Impressed Thought

The Law of Impressed Thought says that every thought or idea impressed on your mind causes a physical reaction. Your thoughts affect your body in profound ways. You don't have to look far to know that this is true. When you are feeling thoughts of stress or anger, your heart races and your respiration changes. When you are worried or anxious, you often have stomach problems. However, it goes far beyond this because the emotions you feel also create hormonal changes in your body. The stronger the emotion, the greater the impact on the body.

A great example of this is when you look at sugary foods and imagine yourself eating them. The subconscious responds to this by lowering your blood sugar in anticipation of the expected sugar intake when you eat it. This in turn just makes you crave it more!

Physical symptoms caused by emotions also tend to create organic changes over time. It is believed that the majority of illnesses are not because of an organic problem in the body. Instead, they are because of a disruption in the nervous system caused by the subconscious mind due to long-term negative emotions. Our minds and our bodies cannot be separated. What affects one will affect the other.

Understanding how your thoughts and emotions affect your physical body is key to creating long-term changes in your body. These long-term changes include controlling cravings, along with losing weight and keeping it off.

3. The Law of Dominant Effect

The Law of Dominant Effect says that the strongest emotion is what will be expressed in your life (and in your body) through the subconscious mind. If you really want to succeed yet have a stronger subconscious fear of failure, the fear of failure will cause you to self-sabotage every time. Likewise, if you really want to lose weight but have a stronger emotional attachment to the lifestyle that is keeping you overweight, your body will not change for any substantial length of time until that attachment is resolved.

4. The Law of Imaginative Effect

The Law of Imaginative Effect says imagination and emotion are more powerful than knowledge when it comes to impacting your subconscious mind. How often do you know what the right thing to do is, but you still find yourself doing what you emotionally want to do because you imagine the good feelings you will receive from it?

Emotional eating is a good example of this. Even though you know sticking to your healthy eating and fitness plan will make you happier in the long run, the emotions produced from imagining how good that cookie will taste wins out every time. The good news is that this law, as you will learn, also provides a solution to the problem.

The subconscious mind cannot differentiate between things that actually happen and things you imagine except to the degree that they are emotionalized (feeling emotion while imagining). This means that if you are able to imagine something in an emotional way, the subconscious mind believes it actually happened.

As you will learn through the *Fat to Fearless*® program, this is one of the keys to providing your subconscious with new evidence about who you are, and then convincing it that you are not an overweight person that cannot lose weight but a thin and healthy person who loves life and loves your body. Once you understand how to do this, the subconscious mind will accept it as true and begin to construct your body and environment to match this new image by changing your habits, behaviors, feelings, and emotions to support what you've imagined.

5. The Law of Expectancy

The Law of Expectancy says that what you expect tends to be realized. Remember the Law of Imaginative Effect says that the subconscious mind acts upon what you imagine. Expecting something to happen is a form of imagining it to happen, just at a slightly lower level of conscious awareness.

When you worry that things are not going your way and you find yourself in an unproductive emotional state, then your fears usually come true. Yet we all know people that seem to be lucky and things always go their way. These people expect good things to happen, and their subconscious sets about creating this outcome for them.

During my almost 20 years of working with weight loss clients, I can tell you that those who struggled for years to lose weight and yo-yoed up and down with various diets did not truly believe that they would be successful. At the conscious level, they tried to give themselves pep talks to believe this, but underneath the surface their doubts about losing the weight and truly keeping it off outweighed their certainty. Subconsciously, they expected they would not lose weight permanently, so they never did.

6. The Law of Repetitive Effect

The Law of Repetitive Effect states that if something is repeated enough, the subconscious mind eventually accepts it as true. This is one of the reasons it is so important to watch your self-talk. Every time you look in the mirror and tell yourself that you are fat or a failure, or that you are never going to lose weight, you program your subconscious mind to make that true for you.

Repetitive actions also influence the subconscious mind. Every time you make a commitment to change your eating habits or exercise but do not follow through, you send a message to the subconscious mind about your true intention. Every time you give in, your subconscious mind supports your true intention and makes it easier to not follow through the next time. Fortunately, the Law of Repetitive Effect can be used to your advantage to reprogram the subconscious mind for permanent weight loss.

7. The Law of Last Experience

The Law of Last Experience says that the last thing we experience about a situation or event tends to be what sticks with us and what we remember most. For example, say you were on a date that you really enjoyed, and your date complimented you many times, but the last thing they said to you was something you thought wasn't flattering. That last comment will color your memory of the entire experience. Had the non-flattering comment been made in the middle of the date, and then followed by the compliments, you would have instead had a more positive feeling about the night when you looked back on it.

This is important to understand when it comes to weight loss. You can make great progress, but then hear one offhand comment from a well-meaning friend or read something discouraging, and that affects your entire view of how well you are doing. Unfortunately, this often causes your emotions to spiral down and leads to emotional eating. This is because you evaluate your progress based on your feeling in that moment instead of what you know to be true about your progress. Since you also know that the subconscious mind responds more to emotion than reason, it is easy to see how not understanding the way these laws work together can lead to self-sabotage.

8. The Law of Subconscious Acceptance

The Law of Subconscious Acceptance tells us that once a belief has been adopted by the subconscious mind as true, it acts on those beliefs until it is replaced by another belief. This law also tells us that the longer an idea stays in your subconscious, the harder it is to change as it is continuously self-reinforced.

Without a program like *Fat to Fearless*® that creates shifts in beliefs at the subconscious level, it is very difficult to change. You can consciously decide that things are going to be different, but until the negative core beliefs you carry in your subconscious are changed, you will always self-sabotage, and you will never succeed.

9. The Law of Diminishing Opposition

The Law of Diminishing Opposition tells us that every thought, action, or suggestion creates less opposition in the subconscious mind to repeating that thought, action, or suggestion in the future.

For example, the first time you talk unkindly to yourself and feel bad about it, you may think, *I can't believe I just thought that about myself*. However, every time you repeat those thoughts, they come easier, seem more true, and are met with less internal opposition.

Every time you tell yourself you are going to work out and don't, it's easier to not follow through the next time. Every time you commit to a healthy eating plan and end up overeating, it gets easier to overeat again.

If you are reading this book, you have probably conditioned yourself to make plans to lose weight and not follow through. Between The Law of Diminishing Opposition and the Law of Repetitive Effect, you have programmed yourself at the subconscious level to not succeed. Fortunately, we will soon use these same laws to turn it all around.

10. The Law of Pain and Pleasure

The Law of Pain and Pleasure says that the subconscious first moves away from pain, and then moves toward pleasure. You will see how important this law is when you learn about creating long-term motivation to not just lose weight but maintain your new weight for a lifetime. For now, understand that the subconscious mind's first priority, before even considering pleasure, is to eliminate pain.

Later, you will learn how the subconscious defines pain, and one thing that is definitely painful to the subconscious is anything that is unknown or inconsistent with its core beliefs. For example, if you believe at the subconscious level that you are a failure and will never succeed, being successful (at losing weight, for example) will be outside of your subconscious comfort zone. Until you change those unconscious beliefs about yourself, your subconscious will work against you achieving the success you want and deserve.

11. The Law of Subconscious Certitude

The Law of Subconscious Certitude is the most important law for you to understand. I frequently call it The Master Law. The Law of Subconscious Certitude states that the subconscious always seeks to make itself right. If you believe things about yourself—such as you are not good enough, you do not deserve to be wealthy, you are destined to be alone, you are a fat person, or any other belief, good or bad—then your subconscious is only too happy to make that come true for you.

You will learn exactly how the subconscious does this, but for now just know that once you have adopted a belief into your subconscious mind, it will make sure that belief shows up in your life. This master law governs your work throughout the rest of the program. Once you truly believe at the subconscious level that you will succeed, that you deserve the body you have always wanted, and you believe you will have it, your subconscious mind will swing into action to ensure that becomes your reality.

As previously mentioned, these 11 Weight Loss Laws of the Mind are the keys to unlocking the power of your subconscious mind. If you have been trying to lose weight while self-sabotaging yourself, then your subconscious has been working against you. By using these 11 laws with the rest of the *Fat to Fearless®* program, you will soon begin to change the self-sabotaging behaviors that have kept you out of those new clothes you've been wanting to buy for the lean body you've been unable, until now, to achieve. You will program yourself for long-term weight loss success.

Now that you understand the laws and the power of the subconscious mind, it's time to learn what the subconscious mind does with all that power. You will learn about core beliefs and how, for much longer than you consciously remember, they have been unconsciously creating your body just as it is right now. To truly change your life at a fundamental level, to go from *Fat to Fearless®*, you must change your core beliefs.

SUMMARY

Key Points

- The Weight Loss Laws of the Mind are a user's manual for how the subconscious mind works. When you understand these laws, you see how your subconscious may have been working against you in your weight loss efforts.

- When you understand the laws, you use them to get your subconscious working for you when losing weight.

What This Has To Do With Weight Loss

The Weight Loss Laws of Mind provide great insight into your subconscious mind. When you understand how to apply these, along with the other skills you'll be learning, you'll be able to have a great deal of control over your behaviors and compulsions. When you understand why certain behaviors cause certain responses from your subconscious, you begin working with your subconscious to make it easier to lose weight and keep it off. When you combine your understanding of the Weight Loss Laws of Mind with the other skills you will learn in the coming chapters, you will truly empower yourself to lose weight easily and change your life.

You Are Ready To Move To The Next Chapter When . . .

- You have a basic understanding of each of the Weight Loss Laws of Mind. At this point, it's not important that you are able to clearly see how each of these laws have affected your ability to lose weight. You will gain more insight as you go through the program. Also, don't feel as if there is any need to memorize these laws. This book will serve as a constant reference as you go through the program.

- You have watched the tutorial video for this chapter and are following the included instructions for actively listening to your Hypnotherapy Audio Sessions (if you have the full *Fat to Fearless®* program).

- You have completed the exercises for this chapter in the Success Guide and Workbook (if you have the full *Fat to Fearless®* program).

PART III

YOUR BELIEFS AND YOUR BODY

CHAPTER 3

THE POWER OF BELIEFS

What do you believe about yourself? The answer to this question is the single most important factor in determining your weight loss success as well as the quality of your entire life.

There are different levels of beliefs. Some beliefs are merely facts about ourselves, such as our name and where we live. Other beliefs are about our capabilities, such as if we believe we will ever become wealthy or if we have what it takes to lose weight and keep it off. But these are not the types of beliefs I'm talking about. I'm talking about beliefs that are so deep, so ingrained into the very nature of who we are, that we call them core beliefs. A core belief is something you believe is true about yourself at a subconscious level, regardless of what anyone else believes. Because the belief is subconscious, you often aren't aware of it and may not even realize it is a belief you have.

Our core beliefs determine our entire lives, including what our bodies look like and whether or not we ever reach our weight loss goals. There are certain core beliefs that tend to always be present in those who chronically fight their weight their whole life. These beliefs usually are similar to *I'm not good enough (or undeserving or not worthwhile)*, with additional beliefs of being *flawed* or *unlovable* mixed in for good measure.

To varying degrees, most of my clients and patients over the years have been conscious that they felt this way about themselves while others had developed coping mechanisms that kept them in denial. If you are reading this book, it is likely that you have struggled with the yo-yo weight cycle much of your life. You are probably asking yourself if you have any of these beliefs and what role they have played in your weight loss struggle. Some of you may realize that these beliefs have been a part of you for as long as you can remember, while others don't quite see it yet or are even resistant to the idea that you believe these things about yourself.

In this book, you're going to learn a lot about the nature of the mind, especially the subconscious mind. When something is subconscious, it means that you are not consciously aware of it. But not realizing it doesn't make it false. The things that we are unconscious of and refuse to believe about ourselves exert more influence and more control in our lives because of their hidden nature. The good news is, because you have been unaware of it, it hasn't been your fault and now you will be able to begin to change these subconscious beliefs that have been holding you back.

If you think you don't have any negative core beliefs, yet you have struggled with weight loss most of your life, then not being able to acknowledge these negative core beliefs is giving them control over your life. In turn, this makes it even harder to change your body in a way that is inconsistent with those beliefs. In the long run, being conscious is always better than being in denial.

Usually the core beliefs that keep us from losing weight are also affecting other areas of our life. They affect our self-esteem and our willingness to take risks, and they keep us in a carefully concealed prison of lowered expectations hidden behind the curtain of what appears to be "realism."

The *Fat to Fearless*® program will show you that weight loss is only the beginning. When you transform the core beliefs that have kept you in your weight loss/weight gain cycle, almost every other area of your life will improve.

This is what is called generative change, where change in one area of your life propagates into other areas. The concept of generative change is at the heart of becoming fearless and living the life of your dreams. Remember, this is not only about losing weight but also about becoming happier than you have ever been before.

In the coming chapters you will learn how core beliefs are formed, how they are self-maintained for a lifetime unless you have intervention at the subconscious level, how to uncover your own core beliefs, and how to begin transforming them into new and positive core beliefs that will empower you to reach your life goals, not just permanent weight loss.

Before moving on to the next chapter, go to the exercise for this chapter in your *Fat to Fearless*® Success Guide and Workbook and complete the exercise. If you don't have the full program with the workbook and videos, I would encourage you to invest in yourself by downloading it from:

www.fattofearless.com

Otherwise, complete the exercise below on your own paper.

EXERCISE: MY THOUGHTS ABOUT BELIEFS

Briefly journal your thoughts on this chapter. Specifically, address how willing you are to see any of the previously mentioned negative beliefs that are common in overweight people in yourself. Openly write about any skepticism you may have so that you can see how it changes as you go through the program and begin to lose weight through subconscious change.

SUMMARY

Key Points

- What we believe about ourselves at a very deep and sub-conscious level is called our "core beliefs."

- Our core beliefs, through mechanisms of the subconscious mind, influence every area of our lives, including our bodies and our ability to lose weight and keep it off.

- While we may know some of our more obvious core beliefs because they exist at the subconscious level, most of us aren't aware of all of our core beliefs.

- The core beliefs that cause us the most difficulty are usually the ones we are least aware of and least want to admit having.

- Your inability to be aware of and admit to these negative core beliefs gives them more power over you.

- The most common negative core beliefs among people who have struggled their whole life with being overweight are: I'm not good enough (or undeserving or not worthwhile), I'm flawed in some way, I'm unlovable.

- Generative change is when change in one area of your life allows you to also make positive changes in other areas of your life.

- The subconscious mind uses your core beliefs as an "operating system" or blueprint for how to construct your life. Remember, one of the primary functions of the subconscious mind is to prove itself right. Because of this, using mechanisms and tools you're going to learn about, you ensure that the experiences you attract into your life, as well as your perception of those experiences, confirm your existing core beliefs.

- In the coming chapters, you will learn how core beliefs are formed, what your core beliefs are, and how to change them to allow you to lose weight and keep it off.

What This Has To Do With Weight Loss

If you have struggled with being overweight your entire life then part of the problem undoubtedly lies in your subconscious mind. This isn't opinion, but fact. If the full processing power of your subconscious mind, along with its ability to control your autonomic nervous system (your metabolism for example) were aligned with your conscious goal of losing weight and keeping it off, it would be almost impossible for you not to succeed.

Whenever the subconscious isn't working to make conscious goals easy to realize, having core beliefs that conflict with these goals are almost always the root of the problem. This is because our core beliefs function as the "operating system" for our subconscious mind. If our subconscious isn't making it easier for us to reach our goals then we must change what's in our subconscious. We must change our core beliefs.

Remember one of the primary functions of the subconscious mind is to prove itself right, nowhere does this apply more than in proving our core beliefs to be true. Specifically, if our core beliefs are that we are in any way "less than," "not good enough," "unattractive," "unlovable," or "unworthy," then being overweight is a great way for our subconscious to prove to us that these things are true.

Once you have transformed your core beliefs to those you deserve to have and keep the body you want, your subconscious will act on these new beliefs to ensure you succeed.

You Are Ready To Move To The Next Chapter When . . .

- You are open to the possibility that core beliefs that you may not be aware of may be playing a significant role in your current and past inability to lose weight and keep it off. At this point, it's okay to be skeptical. In the coming chapters, as you learn more, all of the pieces of how hidden beliefs have affected almost every area of your life will fall into place.

- You have watched the tutorial video for this chapter and are following the included instructions to actively use your Hypnotherapy Audio Sessions (if you have the full *Fat to Fearless®* program).

- You have completed the exercises for this chapter in the Success Guide and Workbook (if you have the full *Fat to Fearless®* program).

CHAPTER 4

HOW CORE BELIEFS ARE FORMED

As a Subconscious Behaviorist and Clinical Hypnotherapist, I have witnessed how core beliefs have influenced and often unconsciously controlled every area of the lives of countless clients. Understanding how core beliefs are formed often helps people understand why they may not be consciously aware of the beliefs they have.

Core beliefs are predominately formed in childhood, usually before the age of ten, and often much younger. It is very easy to understand how core beliefs are formed at such a young age when you understand the nature of the mind and how it works during those early formative years.

You've learned a lot already about the subconscious mind and the rules by which it operates. Now let me introduce you to a psychological equation that has the power to set you free. Once you understand and are able to apply this equation, you will have the ability to change any behavior and achieve success in every area of your life.

EVENTS → BELIEFS → EMOTIONS (resulting from experiences filtered through the beliefs) → SYMPTOMS → REINFORCE YOUR BELIEFS

EVENTS lead to BELIEFS that lead to EMOTIONS that lead to SYMPTOMS that REINFORCE YOUR BELIEFS. Let's look at each step more closely.

Events Lead to Beliefs

We have events that happen in life, and from these events we form certain beliefs. Some examples might be: I'm always going to be alone, I'm not good enough, men/women can't be trusted, people I love leave, I'm unlovable, etc.

Beliefs Lead to Emotions

Once you have these beliefs, you begin constructing your reality around them and filtering your perceptions of events to fit in with what you believe. This obviously creates emotions. If you believe you aren't good enough, or that people you love always leave, that's going to lead to corresponding feelings. Most likely these emotions will be along the lines of sadness, anger, guilt, fear, etc.

Emotions Lead to Symptoms

The natural response to negative emotions is to try to do something to make yourself feel better. Depending upon the environment you were raised in, that may be food, drugs, alcohol, sex, people pleasing, etc. What you use to self-soothe will in part depend upon what was easily available in your childhood environment as well as what you modeled from your caretakers and peers. If you are reading this book, you most likely learned at a young age that food had the ability to make you feel better.

Symptoms Reinforce Core Beliefs

Another principle that determines what you subconsciously choose to self-soothe these negative emotions is that your "drug of choice" will always serve to reinforce the beliefs that created the feelings you're trying to soothe to begin with. In other words, if you believe that you're unlovable and not good enough, you choose food to self-soothe because it makes you overweight (the symptom), and being overweight reinforces your belief that you are unlovable and not good enough. It's a vicious self-reinforcing cycle that keeps you emotionally and physically trapped. *Fat to Fearless®* is about breaking this pattern and creating a new cycle that reinforces positive beliefs about yourself that empower you to lose weight and have the body you want. To do this you must understand a little bit more about how beliefs are formed.

Most of your core beliefs come from events in early childhood. To children, the world is a place of unlimited possibility, and they are well equipped to learn quickly. When I think of my own life, and the lives of all the clients I have worked with, it amazes me how long it takes for us to learn lessons as adults compared to how quickly we learn them as kids.

Children are like sponges and are able to absorb vast amounts of information quickly. One of the best examples of this is children who come from bilingual homes and by the age of eight or younger are fluent in two or more languages. We lose much of this ability later in life.

As adults, we've all had the experience of repeating the same patterns over and over in various areas of our lives ranging from yo-yo weight loss to unhealthy relationships and career choices. Many have been stuck in the same pattern for decades before finally learning what in retrospect seemed like common sense.

To understand what this has to do with core beliefs, we must understand the Critical Gateway. Let's learn why the core beliefs that hold us back are almost always created in childhood and rarely as adults.

Conscious/Subconscious Mind Model

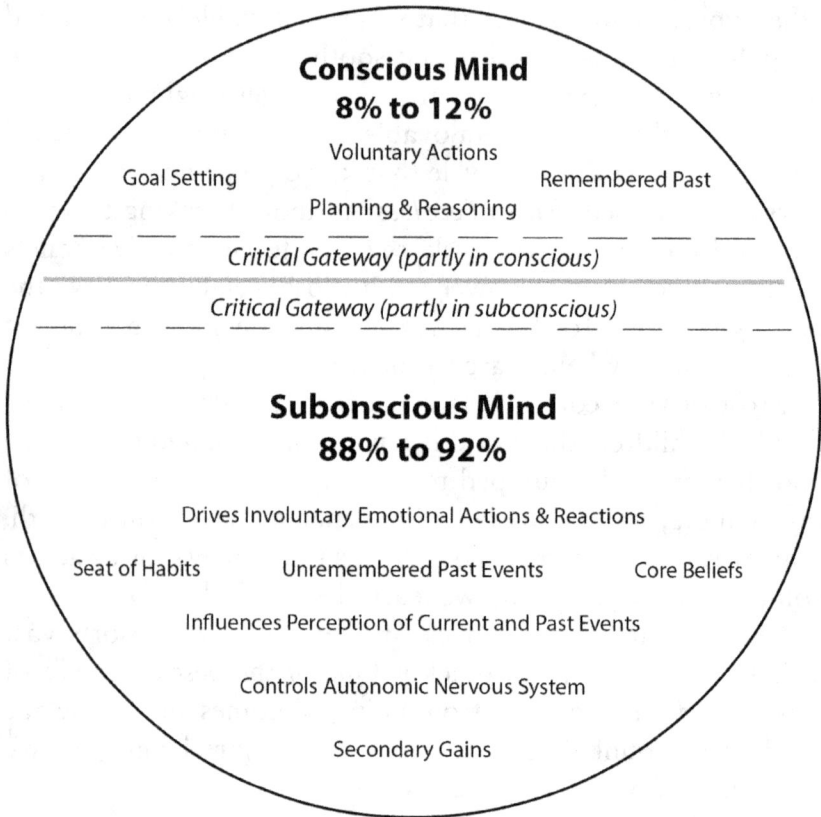

Conscious Mind
8% to 12%

Voluntary Actions

Goal Setting   Remembered Past

Planning & Reasoning

Critical Gateway (partly in conscious)

Critical Gateway (partly in subconscious)

Subonscious Mind
88% to 92%

Drives Involuntary Emotional Actions & Reactions

Seat of Habits   Unremembered Past Events   Core Beliefs

Influences Perception of Current and Past Events

Controls Autonomic Nervous System

Secondary Gains

The Critical Gateway (also called the Critical Factor or Critical Area of the Mind) is located partly in both the conscious and subconscious mind and functions as a filter, a gate keeper, that determines what reaches our subconscious. While we may experience many things in our adult lives that could serve to form our core beliefs or change existing ones, very few of these experiences ever impact the subconscious in a way that affects us deeply enough to produce change. Our preexisting beliefs do not change because the Critical Gateway does not let new and contradicting information reach the subconscious. This has to do with the Law of Subconscious Certitude that you learned earlier which states that the subconscious always seeks to prove itself right.

The job of the Critical Gateway is to compare new information with the beliefs already contained in the subconscious mind and determine if they match. If it is a close enough match, it lets the experience through the filter which allows it to sink into our subconscious. If not, it rejects it, causing it to "bounce off" of our Critical Gateway and never reach the subconscious. By only letting information reach the subconscious that agrees with our preexisting beliefs, it serves to always prove itself right by rejecting any contradictory information as untrue.

This is why young children do not have a Critical Gateway; they have not yet formed the beliefs that serve as a filtering mechanism to determine what is accepted and what is rejected. By default, everything sinks in. This is great for your ability to use the enormous processing capabilities of the subconscious to learn quickly in the early years of life. However, it is less than ideal when, in childhood, experiences cause you to form unhealthy core beliefs that often stay with you for a lifetime.

The Critical Gateway is practically nonexistent in children under the age of 7. Around the ages of 7 to 11, it begins to form and solidify. By the time you are 15 or 16, it is usually fully formed and ready to serve as gatekeeper to the subconscious mind. It then ensures that whatever core beliefs we have formed up to this point remain our core beliefs for the rest of our lives unless we use specific methods of bypassing the Critical Gateway. It does this by rejecting information and experiences that contradict existing core beliefs.

It is rare that our core beliefs shift much in our lifetime because of the Critical Gateway mechanism. However, going through a program like *Fat to Fearless*® that uses proven methods of getting past the Critical Gateway, works to replace unhealthy core beliefs with positive ones by bypassing the Critical Gateway.

It is important to understand that the Critical Gateway is not all bad. Without the Critical Gateway, life would be rather difficult because every new experience and event would have the potential of completely changing your beliefs and the way you view the world. Life would feel like a roller coaster without any clear or stable sense of who you are and what you believe.

Because the Critical Gateway doesn't begin to form until around the ages of 7 to 11, we are able to take advantage of the tremendous processing power of the subconscious mind to learn and develop quickly. However, the downside to this tremendous ability is that all of the information that is going directly into our subconscious is being interpreted with the intellect and emotional maturity of a child.

Would you hire a seven-year-old to run your life? The answer is hopefully a resounding NO, but most of us have a young child's beliefs functioning as the operating system and blueprint for our entire lives. The resulting misinterpretation of childhood events, and what we believe these events mean about us, are often the foundation for the negative core beliefs we carry with us for a lifetime.

My client Jessica, who came to me for weight loss, is an example that helps illustrate how core beliefs that can last a lifetime can be formed early in life. Jessica's example also illustrates how often these beliefs are based on misperceptions inherent in a young child's inability to accurately perceive events in the world around them.

Jessica was four years old, and her sister, Aubrey, had been sick for what seemed like an eternity. While it had actually only been a couple of weeks, children process time differently as they live more in the "now." They also interpret the past, present, and their projected future based on what they are feeling in the moment.

Jessica felt like this was the way things had always been with only a vague awareness that things had been different before. Aubrey being sick was not what troubled Jessica because she didn't quite understand what being sick meant. Not really. Instead, she interpreted it the way all four-year-olds interpret everything—by what it meant to her. What Aubrey's sickness meant to Jessica was that she was getting little to no attention while it seemed like her parents were showering Aubrey with unlimited affection.

In an attempt to reclaim the center of attention, Jessica did the only thing that seemed to have consistently worked in the past, everything she was not supposed to do. It worked, yet not the way that she had hoped. Her parents seemed harsher than usual when correcting her, and they had less interest in consoling her or making up afterward.

This reinforced what Jessica was beginning to believe: they loved Aubrey more. They would tell her things like, "Jessica, how could you do that? Don't you see that Aubrey needs all of my attention right now?" And, "Jessica, Mommy is really too tired for this right now; go play in your room; I need to check on Aubrey." Core beliefs were beginning to form.

It was not long before Jessica noticed Aubrey's absence from the house. Apparently she was in a place called "the hospital" that she remembered as being very much like the doctor's office. A big part of her was very happy that now she would have Mom and Dad to herself.

But this did not go as she hoped either. Mom and Dad frequently left her with the babysitter and spent time with Audrey at the hospital. When they were home, they seemed to show her even less attention than before.

If she were older, this would all make sense because she would understand that her parents were tired and frustrated from working full-time, spending hours at the hospital after work with their sick daughter, all while trying to keep the household running. If she were older, she would have realized that her parents' behavior did not mean that they loved her any less than her sister, and if she were the one sick, they would be doing the exact same thing for her. But she wasn't older, and this was exactly what she was beginning to believe in her four-year-old mind.

She could not understand that if what they told her was true and she didn't need to worry about her sister and that Aubrey was going to be okay, why were they completely neglecting her in favor of Aubrey? In her child's mind, the only conclusion she could come up with was that she was second best and her parents didn't love her, or at least loved her less than Aubrey and less than she wanted. With no Critical Gateway in place at her age, her interpretation of these events went straight into her subconscious.

Things went from bad to worse for Jessica when Aubrey finally came home. Her parents had a homecoming party for her on the day she came back from the hospital. All of their relatives were there, and all of the attention was on Aubrey. They told Aubrey how good she looked, and how great it was to have their beautiful little girl back. Now Jessica was not only second best, but she was not the pretty one either. The core beliefs that formed from these events over the course of about one month were that she was second best, not lovable, and not attractive.

Let's break this down further using our equation:

EVENTS → BELIEFS → EMOTIONS (resulting from experiences filtered through the beliefs) → SYMPTOMS → REINFORCE YOUR BELIEFS

Events

Jessica, a four-year-old girl, had a sister named Aubrey who suffered from an illness for several weeks. Because the mind of a child tends to work more in the "now," this seemed like a much longer period to her. During this time her sister received a lot more attention from her family. The young girl knew her sister was sick, but a four-year-old still processes events based on how they feel in the moment, not based on objective information. She felt that her parents loved her sister more, and that she was only second best.

After a few weeks, the young girl's sister went to the hospital for several days. Her parents, understandably, spent more time at the hospital and left the young girl alone with the babysitter.

She did not understand what was going on, and she felt abandoned. This confirmed her belief that she was not loved as much as her older sister.

When her older sister returned home, even more attention was lavished on her by her parents and other family members. Because her older sister had recovered and no longer looked so pale and sick, everyone told her how good she looked and how beautiful she was. The young girl only noticed that she was not receiving the same attention or compliments about her looks. In her child's mind she reasoned that if she were actually beautiful and they loved her as much as her sister, they would certainly have told her that as much as they were now telling her sister.

Beliefs

From these events, the young girl concluded that she was not good enough, she was second best, and she was unattractive.

Filtering Reality through these beliefs

Once this belief was formed, she filtered all of her experiences through it. The subconscious mind takes beliefs as instructions for what is "true" in the world and ensures our experiences in life conform to that truth. Through the use of the R.A.S. and cognitive distortions (two subconscious mechanisms you will learn about), all of her new experiences were interpreted in ways that were consistent with those beliefs.

During the weeks after her older sister's recovery, the parents once again began showing more attention to the young girl. Unfortunately, the belief was already set in her subconscious, and she thought they were pitying her. From this point forward, all of her experiences were interpreted in a way that continued to build on her misbelief that was based on a child's misperception.

Emotions

After events in life began being filtered through these negative core beliefs, emotions resulted. Emotions of sadness, shame, fear (that she was flawed and not good enough), loneliness, and anger were the result of believing these things about herself.

Symptoms

To help cope with these feelings and avoid dealing directly with them, she developed means of self-soothing these feelings. The type of symptoms we develop are usually based on two things:

1. The path of least resistance or what is easiest based on our environment.

2. The symptom usually creates feedback from our environment that appears to confirm the core belief.

The young girl's family did not practice healthy eating habits. Frequently sweets and other "goodies" were around that her mother used as a reward for good behavior. The young girl learned to use food to make herself feel better.

Reinforces the Belief

Self-soothing her negative emotions with food led to her being overweight, which in turn led to negative feedback about her appearance throughout her life. This reinforced the negative core beliefs she formed during the original event of being unattractive and unlovable.

It Cycles Again

Throughout the course of her life, she tried many diets and fitness programs to lose weight. While she met with short term success, that success didn't change the way she felt about herself long term. Subsequently, it didn't change her need to go back to her only reliable coping mechanism to self-soothe—food.

When Jessica first visited me she knew low self-esteem was a major stumbling block for her life. She related to me an instance that had occurred to her shortly before our first appointment that illustrates the futility of trying to keep weight off without doing the deeper emotional work.

At one point before coming to see me she had managed to lose her excess pounds and reach her goal weight. While she felt better about herself at times, she still thought of herself as second best and not good enough. She thought she was more attractive than when she was overweight, but she was still not attractive *enough*. She was still not lovable. Because she still had the same negative core beliefs, she filtered reality and all of her experiences in the same way to produce the same emotions that she soothed with food regardless of her slimmer body.

At one point during the height of her weight loss she walked into the local mall to shop for shoes. She was wearing tight-fitting clothes that she would never have felt confident enough to wear before she lost weight.

As she entered the mall, she noticed a group of attractive men her age that seemed to be looking at her, and were also joking among themselves. At first she thought that they might be admiring her in a positive way, but within moments she found herself doubting this.

By the time she left the mall, she had convinced herself that they were probably joking about how she thought she was more attractive than she was and didn't look anywhere near good enough to be wearing those clothes. This of course brought up all of those old negative emotions. After multiple incidents like this, she eventually started using food again to feel better and quickly regained the weight.

No matter what you change on the "outside," unless you change your subconscious core beliefs on the "inside," you will always end up producing or believing to be true some flavor of those beliefs. Her perception of this event in the mall was based entirely on the cognitive distortion you will learn about called "mind reading." It had nothing to do with what actually took place. Because her negative core beliefs had not changed about herself, her subconscious filtered the information and distorted her perception to ensure she came to the same conclusions about herself regardless of how much weight she had lost.

Had she walked into that mall having lost the weight while changing her core beliefs to those that supported her in believing she was attractive and good enough, even though every detail of the experience would have been the exact same, she would have had a different interpretation. Most likely, she would have assumed that the young men found her attractive and that was what they were talking about.

I had a very similar event from my own life that also illustrates the concept:

When I was a child, I had formed the core beliefs that I was unattractive and physically inferior. My subconscious, to prove me right, made sure I was always attracted to women who reinforced this belief. Unfortunately my subconscious didn't let me know this in advance and I was often deep into a relationship before I found this out. After the "honeymoon phase," many of my girlfriends would directly or indirectly tell me that they wished I'd had a better body. Sometimes they would even directly compare me to their prior, more athletic, boyfriends.

This caused me a lot of emotional pain, and through a great deal of conscious effort and hard work I finally managed to lose all of my weight. I met Marilyn shortly after having reached my weight loss goal. We hit it off immediately, yet what started out as a very physically passionate relationship seemed to soon fizzle in that department, and I didn't understand why. In my mind I had this great new body that was exactly what the other women I had been in relationships with said they wanted, yet for some reason my new physique did not seem to inspire Marilyn. One night I asked her why her physical attraction to me was declining.

Marilyn explained that while she was attracted to my personality and thought that I was a good-looking guy, I didn't really have the body of the type of guy she was normally attracted to. I was in shock. How could this be? What did she want, Mr. Olympia? She went on to explain.

"I'm just more attracted to guys with more meat on their bones. My dad was overweight and so were my ex-boyfriends. It just makes me feel safe when I can cuddle with them. It's kind of like they're my big teddy bears. With you, I don't feel that. It's a little intimidating too. I feel like I can't have any fat on me because of how you look."

I had changed my body to what was the ideal for the type of women I had attracted in the past, so to prove my belief systems right, my subconscious had to unconsciously drive me to be attracted to a woman who had a preference for overweight men. My body had changed, yet my beliefs hadn't so my subconscious engineered different circumstances to produce the same outcome. Despite my new athletic body, I heard the exact same thing: I am not attracted to you because you are second best.

From my example you can begin to understand why it is crucial to change your core beliefs while changing your body. Even if I could snap my fingers and magically make you be at your goal weight and somehow keep it off, the way you feel about yourself would not change for long. Your subconscious would find a new way to make you feel "bad" about yourself by proving your negative core beliefs true in other ways with a different set of symptoms.

Often, when hearing about circumstances like the one I described from my own life, the question is asked "but how could your subconscious know that she would be attracted to overweight men?" While this could also be a book within itself, it's easy to grasp why we can't grasp this when you remember the level at which the subconscious mind is operating.

In any given moment your subconscious is instantaneously processing 500 times more information beyond what you are even aware of and retaining it for life. It is also cross-referencing that information with everything that's been stored in your subconscious since the womb. From this storehouse of information and awareness it is able to develop limitless pro-files of people, personality types, circumstances, and projected outcomes and intuitively come to conclusions about this infor-mation. If we were capable of consciously understanding this, then it wouldn't be subconscious.

Events that form negative beliefs about ourselves are some-times legitimately traumatic, as in the case of childhood physi-cal and sexual abuse or true emotional neglect and psychologi-cal trauma. Other times, like in Jessica's case, they are seem-ingly small events that became major turning points in your life because of how you interpreted them based on your limited emotional and intellectual understanding as a child.

Beliefs can be formed as a result of all or any of our child-hood experiences and are usually a combination of all of them. Your parents, school teachers, classmates, relatives, and any-one else of significance in your formative years can play a role in shaping what you believe about yourself and the world you live in.

It is important to understand that during these early years the subconscious is eager to form what will become your core beliefs. This is because your core beliefs act as an operating system for your life. They help you evaluate what is true and what is not, help you determine the actions you take or do not take, as well as subtly serve as guidelines for your thoughts and opinions.

Without beliefs, the world is a chaotic and unpredictable place. Your beliefs about yourself and the world provide a sense of stability, an understanding of how things are. If given the choice between having no beliefs and having negative ones, you will always choose negative beliefs. If you were a com-puter, would you want no operating system at all or a faulty one that at least allowed you to perform basic functions?

Listed on the next page are the most common core beliefs I have found present in my clients who have been unable to lose weight and keep it off.

- I am not good enough.
- I am unlovable.
- I am alone.
- I am not safe.
- I will always be abandoned.
- Being intimate means being vulnerable.
- If people get to know the real me, they will not like me.
- Sex and being sexual is bad.
- I am ugly.
- I am out of control.
- I'm a loser.

While these core beliefs are most common in chronically overweight clients, this list is by no means exhaustive. Soon you will uncover your own core beliefs that are holding you back from having the body and life you want.

Events you experienced as a child, without your adult mind to analyze and evaluate, are frequently misinterpreted and form negative core beliefs. To understand how this affects your ability to lose weight, you need to add an important principle to your understanding of how the subconscious mind works, and understand how it operates with the Law of Subconscious Certitude.

The subconscious mind interprets core beliefs as instructions for what is true and "right." The Law of Subconscious Certitude says that the subconscious mind always seeks to prove itself right. To do this, it constructs your life using your core beliefs as a blueprint.

When you understand the way these two important principles work together, it quickly becomes apparent why you want to uncover negative core beliefs and transform them into positive ones. It also becomes apparent how and why core beliefs often play themselves out through weight issues and other self-destructive behaviors.

If I believe the following—I am unlovable, not good enough, will probably end up alone, or being intimate means I am unsafe and vulnerable and leads to being hurt or abandoned— my subconscious mind will prove that those things are true. It does this by engineering circumstances and urging me toward behaviors that reinforce those beliefs. It also skews your interpretation of events in a way that also reaffirms the negative beliefs. (Sabotaging your weight loss is a great way to prove any or all of these beliefs true!)

Ultimately, what you believe about yourself and the world is what comes to pass. You might know people who frequently end up in the same type of limiting or destructive situation no matter how much they consciously say they will never do it again. That is their subconscious acting according to their core beliefs to override what their conscious mind wants.

For example, have you ever noticed how when someone believes *all men cheat* or *all women are unfaithful*, that they always seem to be cheated on in every relationship they are in? Or the person who believes that there are no opportunities to improve their career never seems to get that new job offer, while someone else right next to them with seemingly less experience and less going for them is promoted? This is because of the difference in what they believe and how their subconscious acts on those beliefs to create self-fulfilling outcomes.

As you go through the *Fat to Fearless*® program, you will come to understand how these core beliefs function in your life on every level, how they work to specifically make you overweight, and why every diet, fitness regimen, or weight loss program will never succeed until you heal these unhealthy beliefs by transforming them into ones that support you in achieving the body and life you want.

If you subconsciously believe that you are unlovable, not good enough, or unattractive, what better way does your subconscious mind have of proving this to be true than by making you overweight and ensuring you always keep that weight on. In our society, the more being fit and slim becomes the standard for beauty, and being physically attractive becomes more important through the images we see on TV, film, and in magazines, the more likely it is that if we have negative core beliefs, our subconscious mind is going to use body fat to prove to us that those negative beliefs are correct.

But we are getting ahead of ourselves. You now understand how negative beliefs are formed and you know that the subconscious mind works to make itself right and to prove these beliefs true. You also have a basic understanding of how and why being overweight is one of the primary ways it does this. But once negative core beliefs are formed, why do they not change when you have positive experiences in life? If we think back to the example of my client Jessica, why after her sister got better and she started getting positive attention from her parents again did it not counteract the prior negative experiences? To answer this question you must understand how these negative beliefs are maintained and preserved in your mind after they are formed.

EXERCISE: CONSCIOUS BELIEF RECALL

Many of the events that form the basis of our core beliefs we can't actively remember, however that's not always the case.

1. In your *Fat to Fearless*® Success Guide and Workbook, or on your own paper, list as many significant events as you can consciously recall before the age of 10.

2. Write down how these events made you feel and what beliefs you think may have formed as a result.

3. Assuming you are correct, and you did form these beliefs from these events, list all the ways you think it has affected you throughout your life.

Forgiveness and Blame

Part of your *Fat to Fearless*® program includes understanding your own life story both as you currently see it, and through new eyes as you begin to uncover your own limiting core beliefs. It's important to understand that this is not about blaming those in your past that you feel wronged you, but about taking responsibility for your life and rewriting the beliefs those childhood experiences created. Blaming others disempowers you. When you understand this process, you also understand that everyone in your life, whether you cast them as victims, villains, or heroes, were simply doing the best they could with the available psychological resources they had at the time.

One of the benefits of resolving your negative core beliefs is eliminating what gave them so much power: your negative judgment of others and how they treated you. By doing this you stop maintaining a victim mentality. Without these negative core beliefs, you no longer hold onto judgment and are free to see people as they are, doing their best with their own circumstances. This freedom paves the way for acceptance and love.

If you were truly wronged or abused, forgiveness doesn't mean saying what was done was "okay." What it means is that you are no longer putting your own active life energy in the present into preserving negative feelings around past events.

The truth is you cannot truly love yourself and hate your past at the same time because the past is what made you who you are, and who you are now actively working to become. As you go through this process, remember that true forgiveness involves no one but you and is the act of setting yourself free from the past so you can move forward in the present.

SUMMARY

Key Points

- Our subconscious interprets our beliefs as a blueprint for how to construct our lives.

- Core beliefs are typically formed from early childhood events.

- An important equation to understanding how beliefs are formed, and then how those beliefs lead to symptoms such as emotional eating, weight gain, and self-sabotage is:

  EVENTS → BELIEFS → EMOTIONS → SYMPTOMS → BELIEF REINFORCEMENT

- We always choose activities to self-soothe that create symptoms that reinforce the core beliefs that created the feelings we are trying to make feel better to begin with. For example, if our core beliefs are that we are unlovable, not good enough, and unattractive, we may choose food to self-soothe because the resulting symptom (being overweight) reinforces our core belief that we are unlovable, not good enough, and unattractive.

- Another example might be that if you had the core belief that you would always be abandoned, you might choose drugs to self-soothe because the resulting behavior might create circumstances that made it difficult for others to stand by you.

- Core beliefs are usually formed in childhood, usually before the age of 10, and often younger.

- The reason core beliefs are easily formed in childhood is that the Critical Gateway, which acts as a filter for what is allowed to enter the subconscious mind, hasn't yet formed. Because of this, it's easier for children to form new beliefs because of how easily new experiences reach the subconscious.

- Often, these beliefs are negative because as children we don't have the maturity or intellect to accurately perceive what's actually happening. This, coupled with the child-hood tendency to personalize everything, often leads to negative beliefs about our value and worth.

- It is rare that our core beliefs change much throughout our lives because the Critical Gateway only allows information into our subconscious that confirms our already existing beliefs. New, more positive experiences, are typically dismissed and have little impact on what we truly believe about ourselves or the world at the deepest levels.

- The Critical Gateway isn't "bad." The Critical Gateway maintains your positive core beliefs as well as your negative ones. Like all the mechanisms of the subconscious mind it operates impartially by a set of rules. When you understand these rules you can begin making them work for you.

- Unless you have done transformational work at the subconscious level, most of us unknowingly have the beliefs we formed as young children running and often sabotaging our adult lives.

What This Has To Do With Weight Loss

Lifelong struggles with weight issues are one of the ways our negative core beliefs manifest in our lives. One of the hardest things about accepting this is that we often have trouble believing we actually have these negative core beliefs. Often, in our conscious mind, we feel as if we believe the opposite. When you understand the way the subconscious mind works, you know the outcomes of our lives have their roots in a subconscious template. It's not possible for us to behave in ways that are harmful to us (like emotional eating and being overweight) and fully love ourselves at the subconscious level.

It often helps people accept that these negative core beliefs are present in their subconscious when they understand how they are formed. When you realize these beliefs came from childhood, often from events you may not remember, or events that seem insignificant in your adult memory, it's easier to understand how they came to be present without you consciously being aware of them.

Transforming your negative core beliefs to positive ones that support you is absolutely necessary to losing weight and keeping it off. Changing these core beliefs requires accepting they are there and actively working to replace them with better ones. Realizing that many of the beliefs that run your life were formed with the intellect and emotional maturity of a child underscores the importance of the work we are doing together.

You Are Ready To Move To The Next Chapter When . . .

You have a basic understanding that events lead to beliefs—which lead to emotions—which lead to symptoms—which lead to a reinforcement of the beliefs. Specifically, you understand:

- Events, usually from childhood, lead to the development of our beliefs.

- Negative emotions you use food to soothe are a result of experiencing life through your negative core beliefs.

- Using food to self-soothe these emotions leads to being overweight which just reinforces your negative beliefs about yourself.

- You have a strong understanding of why using food to feel better is a vicious cycle that keeps you emotionally and physically trapped.

- You have watched the tutorial video for this chapter and are following the included instructions to actively use your Hypnotherapy Audio Sessions (if you have the full *Fat to Fearless*® program).

- You have completed the exercises for this chapter in the Success Guide and Workbook (if you have the full *Fat to Fearless*® program).

CHAPTER 5

WHY BELIEFS ARE HARD TO CHANGE

You have learned how negative core beliefs are formed and how your subconscious mind takes those beliefs as instructions for how to create your life. Now let's look deeper at why it is so hard to change those beliefs on your own.

You probably know people who are self-help junkies. They read every book they can and try every promising new program with the hope of changing their lives. More often than not, their hope for lasting change falls short of the results they actually get. Why is this?

The reason so many people fail to change their lives significantly is that they only work to create change at the conscious level and do not create subconscious change. The exercises, programs, and techniques they try only work at this superficial level of awareness. They are never able to change their unconscious belief systems because the subconscious has very powerful tools to safeguard and protect those core beliefs so that they don't change, thus always proving those beliefs right. Those beliefs and your inability to change them is the real source of the problem.

At first, the idea that your subconscious is trying to keep you from changing your negative core beliefs may make it seem as if your subconscious is actively against you, but this is not true. The subconscious mind is impartial. Your subconscious doesn't make value judgments about what is right or wrong. It functions by a specific set of rules, many of which you have already learned, and does its job based on those rules. Much like a computer only executes the program it is given, your subconscious only acts on the programming it has received. As you've learned, most of that programming comes from your early life experiences.

A computer would have a hard time doing its job if its internal components were constantly being changed and rewired. So too would your subconscious have trouble doing its job of keeping you safe and functional in the world if your core beliefs were always being changed. To continue with our metaphor, this is why part of the design of a computer includes screws and mechanisms to keep its parts in place as well as an outer casing to protect those same internal components from its environment. Just like that computer, your subconscious mind has mechanisms in place to protect its internal components from your environment. Let's begin learning about the "mechanisms" your subconscious mind uses to protect its "components," your core beliefs.

If you want to rewire that computer, you need to know how to open the casing and learn where all the screws and brackets are that keep everything where it needs to be. If you want to change your core beliefs, you need to have a similar understanding of what your subconscious mind uses to hold your core beliefs in place.

The first step in the process of changing your negative core beliefs into positive ones is to understand why those beliefs have been so hard to change on your own. The second step is using that knowledge to bypass these subconscious defense mechanisms so that you can rewrite your programming and change your core beliefs so that your subconscious actually works with you to help you achieve the body you have always wanted.

Here are three important tools of the subconscious mind that it uses to keep your existing beliefs from changing despite your conscious desire to do so.

1. The Critical Gateway

You've already been introduced to the Critical Gateway, the gatekeeper between your conscious and subconscious mind that filters out information and experiences that contradict what is already in your subconscious. You will gain a deeper understanding of the Critical Gateway to prepare you for learning how to bypass it so you can consciously program your subconscious for success.

2. The Reticular Activating System (R.A.S.)

The R.A.S. is a biological part of your brain, and it determines what pieces of information you become consciously aware of and which information is sent straight to your subconscious mind.

The bad news is that your R.A.S. may not even bring to your conscious awareness the information and experiences you need to help install new and healthy beliefs. The good news is that you can program your R.A.S. to be a life-affirming search engine, always scanning for proof that the positive beliefs you want are actually the ones that are true for you.

3. The Inner Critic

The Inner Critic is perhaps the most unpleasant tool the subconscious uses to keep your existing beliefs in place. It is unpleasant because it also keeps you feeling emotionally bad in the process. The Inner Critic is that negative voice in your head that judges you as "bad" or "wrong" for all the things you do that you believe you "should not" do, and the things that you do not do that you believe you "should." Defeating and transforming this unpleasant voice is not only an important part of changing your negative core beliefs, but is also key to ending emotional eating and improving your overall happiness.

These three subconscious mechanisms—the Critical Gateway, the R.A.S., and the Inner Critic—work together to ensure that your current beliefs do not change. You can change your core beliefs, however, if you know the formula to bypass the Critical Gateway, reprogram your R.A.S., and transform your Inner Critic in to a supportive ally. When you do this you will be reprogramming your subconscious for weight loss success.

It is now time to look under the hood of these three "new-belief busters" so that you can learn the formula to get them working for you instead of against you as you go from *Fat to Fearless*®.

SUMMARY

Key Points

- The reason that most people never succeed in creating any type of real and long-lasting change using self-help material is that they are only working at the conscious level.

- To create any type of real and lasting change you must work at the subconscious level to change your core beliefs.

- Without using a program like *Fat to Fearless*® it is hard to change your core beliefs because the Critical Gateway prevents new information that contradicts those beliefs from reaching the subconscious. This is part of the subconscious' mechanism designed to always prove itself right.

- The three primary mechanisms the subconscious mind uses to hold your existing beliefs in place and keep them from easily changing are the:

  - Critical Gateway
  - Reticular Activating System (R.A.S.)
  - Inner Critic

- When you understand the formula to bypass these subconscious defense systems, you can reprogram your subconscious for weight loss success.

What This Has To Do With Weight Loss

Losing weight and keeping it off requires changing your core beliefs to ones that support you toward that goal. To be able to change your core beliefs you must understand the mechanisms of the subconscious that work against you so you can begin to make them work for you. Everything you are now learning, and will learn as we get deeper into the program, will be applied to allow you to do exactly that.

You Are Ready To Move To The Next Chapter When . . .

- You understand the primary reason most people fail to create permanent change or lasting results when attempting self-help programs is they are only working at the conscious level.

- You understand the importance of working at the subconscious level to change your core beliefs.

- You are prepared to learn more about how the subconscious mind uses the Critical Gateway, the Reticulated Activating System, and the Inner Critic to keep you from easily changing your core beliefs.

- You have watched the tutorial video for this chapter and are following the included instructions to actively use your Hypnotherapy Audio Sessions (if you have the full *Fat to Fearless*® program).

CHAPTER 6

THE CRITICAL GATEWAY

The Critical Gateway is the first of three important tools of the subconscious mind that it uses to keep your existing beliefs from changing despite your conscious desire to do so.

If you've struggled your entire life to lose weight and have never succeeded because of a combination of emotional eating, self-sabotage, and lack of willpower, then the root of the problem is in your subconscious. Specifically, the problem is negative core beliefs about yourself and what you deserve that are driving the behaviors that keep your overweight.

The primary reason your core beliefs do not change once they are formed is because the Critical Gateway guards the entrance to the subconscious mind against any information that comes from new experiences that contradict your preexisting beliefs. These core beliefs keep you overweight.

Understanding how the Critical Gateway works is key to learning how to make the gate open so that new ideas and information—designed to create new, positive, weight loss-reinforcing core beliefs—can reach the subconscious. On the next page is a review of the Critical Gateway.

1. The Critical Gateway begins to form around age seven and is usually solidified by our early-teen years.

2. The Critical Gateway is a judgment-based filter that checks to see if new information is compatible with your existing beliefs. Judgment is the key, "facts" have little value.

3. If the new information is not compatible with your existing beliefs, then it is rejected. If it is consistent with your existing beliefs, then it is allowed to pass into the subconscious. In your subconscious, it affects you on a deeper level and confirms and reinforces the beliefs you already have.

4. Once formed, the Critical Gateway makes it hard to change our core beliefs without using specific techniques to bypass it and reach the subconscious mind so that new information can create new beliefs.

So why does the Critical Gateway make it so hard to change your existing core beliefs? Because if information comes in through new experiences that contradicts your current core beliefs, it has no choice but to reject it or risk compromising your subconscious mind's function of keeping you safe by limiting your beliefs to the ones that it knows has kept you alive and functional up to this point.

Remember, the subconscious is about 90% of our mental functioning. Without producing change at the subconscious level, the 10% that compromises the conscious mind is just left spinning its wheels and swearing that this next attempt to lose weight and keep it off is going to be different.

Since, thanks to the Critical Gateway, the experiences that impact your subconscious are ones that confirm what you already believe about yourself, the deck is stacked against you when trying to reprogram your subconscious, which is absolutely necessary to create a lasting life-change like permanent weight loss.

It is easy to find examples of the Critical Gateway working all around us. We can all relate to the friend that has low self-esteem. No matter how many times they receive compliments that should counteract the negative beliefs about themselves or their abilities, these compliments just seem to bounce off. However, let them receive the slightest criticism and it seems to sink in and have a profound impact, sometimes for days. This is the Critical Gateway at work.

Let's say your friend Mary has the core beliefs that she is not good enough and is unattractive. Mary has been on a diet and losing weight, although not as quickly as she would like. One morning you give her a compliment about how good she looks.

This compliment then hits the Critical Gateway, which in turn says to the subconscious mind, *Hey, we were just told that we were attractive—is this true?* The subconscious mind checks with Mary's existing core beliefs and answers back, *No, we believe we are not good enough and we are unattractive.*

The Critical Gateway then views the compliment as not only untrue, but a direct threat to the subconscious mind's function of proving its existing beliefs correct. The Critical Gateway then rejects the compliment. Because it never reached the subconscious, the compliment is quickly dismissed, and any momentary positive effect it had on your friend Mary, if there was any at all, is gone within moments, having no true impact at all on what Mary believes about herself.

However, let's say that when you saw Mary you were not a particularly good friend and instead of complimenting her, you pointed out that she still had a lot of weight to lose and didn't look very good yet. When this information reaches her Critical Gateway, it turns to ask the subconscious mind if it is true that she doesn't look very good. Her subconscious mind would have responded, *Yes, this is consistent with our core beliefs that we are still not good enough and unattractive.*

The Critical Gateway would then allow your words to sink straight into her subconscious. She takes in the negative words completely, allows them to impact her emotionally at a subconscious level, and probably would not get over it for days, all the while repeating your negative words in her mind. When she then turned to food to feel better and regained some of her lost weight, her subconscious would then have proved itself right by accumulating even more evidence to prove her core beliefs true.

Your Critical Gateway does not actually "speak" to your subconscious any more than your computer's hard drive "speaks" to its monitor, but this metaphor helps to better understand the way they interact. Understanding the way they interact helps us make sense of why different things may impact us in different ways based on what we believe about ourselves.

Another example from my own life shows the Critical Gateway at work:

Many years ago I was hired as a consultant for a fitness company to profile the motivations of their target customers. As part of the research I staffed one of their booth's at a very large women's expo event. This was during yet another time where I had lost my excess weight and had yet to regain it.

Across from our display was the booth for Estée Lauder Cosmetics. Because of the high profile nature of the show, they had staffed the event with beautiful women to serve as their spokesmodels.

It was a two-day event, and at the end of the first day one of the women from the Estée Lauder group approached me. She told me that the women had been talking about me and she wanted me to know that they all found me very attractive. Initially, I was very flattered, as it was exactly the sort of thing I needed to hear to help offset the negative beliefs I carried around from childhood of being unattractive and second best. It felt very good, almost unbelievable that these beautiful women would think this about me. Very soon, it did become unbelievable.

Despite many positive experiences in my adult life like this one that countered my negative subconscious programming, my subconscious mind wouldn't allow me to accept their compliment. Within a short time I convinced myself that they probably didn't mean it, and they were just being nice. By the next day I had convinced myself that they were probably making fun of the ugly guy working the fitness booth and were just amusing themselves at my expense.

It was only in retrospect, after healing my own inner mind, that I could look back on this and dozens of similar events in my life and realize what had happened. Because they were inconsistent with my existing beliefs, my Critical Gateway didn't allow these experiences to effect me at the subconscious level where they could actually change how I felt about myself.

Since most all of us have core beliefs we would like to change, it would be easy to think of the Critical Gateway as something that is more negative than positive, something we wish we didn't have. While it is true the Critical Gateway can make it difficult to change beliefs, it also serves to protect positive beliefs.

All of us are a combination of positive and negative beliefs that play out in our lives. While we may feel bad about ourselves in some areas, there are other areas where we have confidence and do well. It is as hard for new incoming information to change our positive beliefs, as it is to change our negative beliefs.

For example, one of my core beliefs is that I am good with people and understanding the mind and what motivates people's behavior. When I began my career as a Clinical Hypnotherapist, I didn't have the knowledge, skill, and experience that now allows me to have the high success rate I have with all my clients. Yet, because I had the core belief that I had the skills that would allow me to become a great therapist, I did not allow myself to quit or become discouraged in the early years when a client was not getting the results they wanted.

I believed I had the core skills necessary to be a great therapist and simply took failure as feedback that I used to learn and grow and become who I am today. My Critical Gateway did not allow negative experiences in this area to change my positive beliefs anymore than it would allow my negative beliefs to be changed by contradictory experiences.

You can begin to see how the Critical Gateway is not good or bad, but only a part of the way your mind functions. I can't stress this enough: To change your core beliefs, you must reach the subconscious, and to reach the subconscious, you must bypass the Critical Gateway that stands guard.

The Critical Gateway is a powerful component of how existing negative beliefs are maintained in spite of life giving you positive evidence to the contrary. After learning about the other subconscious mechanisms that work to hold your existing beliefs in place, you will learn to overcome them, including how to overcome the limitations imposed by the Critical Gateway.

To begin to see how your Critical Gateway impacts your experience of life, complete the following exercise in the Success Guide and Workbook. If you don't have the full program with the workbook and videos, I would encourage you to invest in yourself by downloading it from www.fattofearless.com. Otherwise, complete the exercise below on your own paper.

EXERCISE: MY CRITICAL GATEWAY

1. List three experiences where someone paid you a compliment or you received praise for something that you dismissed and/or it had little positive impact on you.

   Once you have listed your three positive experiences, write down what you told yourself about them. How did you minimize them?

2. List 3 negative experiences where someone said something derogatory, or you received criticism for something that really affected you.

   Once you have listed your 3 negative experiences, write down what you told yourself about them. Why do you believe they bothered you to the degree they did?

3. Write down, based on the above, how you believe your Critical Gateway may have shaped how you perceived each of the experiences based on beliefs you have about yourself. Even if it doesn't "feel true" at this point that you have a Critical Gateway that functions in this way, hypothesize based on what you have learned so far "as if" it's true. Remember, not consciously being aware of these things doesn't mean it's not actually the case. This will become more clear as you continue through the program.

Next, lets take a deeper look at the R.A.S., Reticular Activating System, which may be keeping you from even seeing the opportunities that present themselves every day for you to change your mind and body.

SUMMARY

Key Points

- To change your core beliefs you must convince your subconscious that the new beliefs that you want are true. To do this, new information that contradicts your old beliefs and reinforces the new ones must reach the subconscious. For this to happen, you must get the Critical Gateway to open.

- The Critical Gateway is one of the mechanisms of the subconscious mind that preserves your existing beliefs and thus serves the subconscious mind's function of always proving itself right.

- Once formed, the Critical Gateway makes it hard to change our core beliefs without using specific techniques to open the gate and reach the subconscious mind so that new information can create new beliefs.

- The Critical Gateway begins to form around age seven and is usually solidified by our early-teen years.

- The Critical Gateway is a judgment-based filter that checks to see if new information is compatible with your existing beliefs. Judgment is the key, facts have little value.

- If the new information is not compatible with your existing beliefs, it is rejected. If it is consistent with your existing beliefs, then it is allowed to pass into the subconscious. In your subconscious, it affects you on a deeper level and confirms and reinforces the beliefs you already have.

- When you receive compliments that go against your core beliefs, they quickly bounce off the Critical Gateway and have little lasting effect on how you feel, either emotionally in the moment or about yourself in any lasting way. However, if you receive a criticism that is consistent with your negative core beliefs, your Critical Gateway allows it to reach your subconscious, and it can bother you for days. This is why your experiences in life always feel as if they are confirming what you already believe at the deepest levels.

- The Critical Gateway is impartial; it preserves our positive core beliefs as well as our negative core beliefs. Once you change your beliefs to positive ones, it will serve to safeguard those and ensure they don't easily revert back to their negative counterparts.

What This Has To Do With Weight Loss

The Critical Gateway is one of the primary mechanisms that make it difficult to change your core beliefs. Because of the way the Critical Gateway functions, we tend to ignore, minimize, or dismiss any information that contradicts what we already believe about ourselves at the deepest level. Much of the time, this information could make it easier for us to lose weight and keep it off. To change your core beliefs to new and healthy ones that support permanent weight loss, you have to get your new programming past the Critical Gateway. The information you learned in this chapter will be used further in to the program to help you do that.

You Are Ready To Move To The Next Chapter When . . .

- You understand how the Critical Gateway works to keep you from easily changing your existing core beliefs.

- You have watched the tutorial video for this chapter and are following the included instructions to actively use your Hypnotherapy Audio Sessions (if you have the full *Fat to Fearless*® program).

- You have completed the exercises for this chapter in the Success Guide and Workbook (if you have the full *Fat to Fearless*® program).

CHAPTER 7

THE R.A.S.

The R.A.S. is the second of those three important tools of the subconscious mind used to keep your existing beliefs from changing.

The Critical Gateway does not have a physical location in the brain because it is a psychological construct. The Reticular Activating System (R.A.S), however, is a set of connected nuclei that connects our brain stem with our cortex. While the R.A.S. has many functions, ranging from the regulation of sleep patterns to regulating various senses in the body, it is also responsible for filtering incoming information to determine what is brought to conscious awareness and what is shuffled into the subconscious.

We have already learned that the conscious mind can only process about 40 bits of incoming information per second as compared to the ability of the subconscious to process 20,000 bits per second. What we have not discussed is how much information actually comes into our brain and needs processing. If we only took in through our senses 40 bits per second of incoming information, then our conscious mind would be able to process all incoming information. Our subconscious mind's processing ability would be irrelevant.

An article in *Current Biology* (July 2006) by Judith McLean and Michael A. Freed from the University of Pennsylvania School of Medicine, and Ronen Segev and Michael J. Berry III from Princeton University, suggests that the human retina alone transmits data to the brain at the rate of 10 million bits per second. That is just our eyes. Now add to that the incoming information from our hearing, tasting, smelling, and touch, and you can see how we take in an incredible amount of information far beyond what the conscious mind can even begin to deal with. Out of all those millions of bits of information, it is the R.A.S. that determines which 40 bits goes to conscious awareness and what is sent directly to the subconscious.

The R.A.S. determines what information is brought to your conscious attention. If you have seen children playing on the playground with their mothers nearby, you have seen an example of this. There may be dozens of children playing on the playground, all in various stages of fun and distress as they fall, occasionally fight, and do all the things that children do when they play together. Yet despite how many children are playing at once or how much noise they are making or how involved the mother is in conversation, the slightest cry from *her child and her child alone* is instantly recognized. She has her R.A.S. to thank for this as it has been programmed to scan and filter all incoming bits of information coming in through her five senses and should any one of these bits indicate her child is in distress of any kind, that information is sent straight to the conscious mind to be immediately acted upon.

Another example of this is our ability to immediately distinguish the sound of our name spoken in a crowded room where everyone is talking at once. The R.A.S. scans all incoming sounds, and should your name be mentioned, it is immediately brought to your conscious awareness. Without the R.A.S., we would be completely lost amidst a sea of incoming data, unable to consciously sort it fast enough to act on the things that need our immediate attention.

It is easy to understand why situations dealing with safety and direct attention are important enough for the R.A.S. to bring to conscious awareness, but what about the rest of the information that could help us change our core beliefs and, among other things, lose weight and keep it off? When it comes to this information, how does the R.A.S. determine what we consciously need to know?

As a survival mechanism, the R.A.S. is hard-wired to bring immediate threats or danger to our attention. These threats can be real or imagined.

A tiger in the bushes, for example, is a real danger. Phobias, however, are often imagined dangers. Katsaridaphobia, the fear of roaches, is an imagined fear of something that is not life-threatening. Your R.A.S scans for any sign of roaches because *you believe* they pose a danger. The R.A.S. filters information according to what you believe at both the conscious and the subconscious level.

The tools that the subconscious mind uses to preserve your core beliefs are powerful. Anything that contradicts your existing beliefs is often sent directly to your subconscious mind by the R.A.S. before you are even aware of it. Now let's look at how this pertains to weight loss.

Let's say you believe people "like you" are not able to lose weight. One day you are visiting with your family while the TV is on, and a news segment talks about a medical breakthrough for people "like you" to lose weight and keep it off. However, you don't notice the news segment because your R.A.S. did not consider it important because it wasn't in alignment with your existing beliefs. Because it was not important, your R.A.S did not send it to your conscious mind and instead you paid attention to all of the other noise, conversations, and distractions in the room.

The R.A.S. has a tendency to filter out of conscious awareness things that do not support your existing core beliefs. Had you already gone through the *Fat to Fearless*® program and transformed your subconscious beliefs about your ability to lose weight, you probably would have immediately keyed in on that news segment despite the distraction of family. Your R.A.S. would have been scanning for information that proved there was a way for you to reach your weight goals.

The R.A.S. does this in all areas of your life. It seeks out information that proves what you truly believe at the deepest level. If you believe there are no opportunities in your field for a job, there could be a conversation taking place right next to you about someone looking for someone just like you, and you may not even notice it. The catch-22 is that even if you did hear it, because finding the perfect job in this way contradicts your core belief that there are no opportunities, it would probably just bounce off your Critical Gateway. You would dismiss it as too good to be true.

This is an example of why it is so important you use a method of transforming your subconscious that simultaneously addresses all the ways you may be sabotaging yourself. They will all work together against you unless you learn how to overcome them and reprogram your subconscious to work for you instead.

If you believe you are not good enough, unattractive, losing weight is difficult, that you hate exercise, or have any other core beliefs that have interfered with your ability to lose weight and keep it off, the R.A.S. ensures that the majority of information that would contradict those beliefs, that would help you to see that those things are not true, never reaches your conscious awareness. Likewise, it ensures that every experience or piece of information that confirms your negative beliefs sticks out like a sore thumb and is easily noticed.

If you do consciously notice things that contradict your existing beliefs, they are quickly rejected by the Critical Gateway, never reaching the subconscious mind, and never having a positive effect. It is the ultimate one-two punch that often keeps people trapped in belief systems that have kept them overweight and caught in the yo-yo cycle of losing and gaining weight most of their lives.

At this point, you may be having a couple of reactions to what you have learned so far. The first reaction is a new understanding of why you struggled to lose weight your entire life. The second reaction is a feeling of discouragement because you feel as if your own subconscious mind is working against you. Take heart, because everything that has worked against you will soon work for you. All of these mechanisms of the mind will soon be helping you lose weight and keep it off.

Once you change your negative core beliefs, your Critical Gateway ensures that you keep them, while your R.A.S. scans your environment for information that proves these new positive beliefs are true. Before long it will continuously bring supporting evidence to your attention.

Complete the following exercise in the Success Guide and Workbook. If you don't have the full program with the workbook and videos, I would encourage you to invest in yourself by downloading it from www.fattofearless.com. Otherwise, complete the exercise below on your own paper:

EXERCISE: WHAT DO I NOTICE?

1. List as many experiences as you can think of where you have overheard conversations in a noisy environment, and answer the following questions:

   What about this conversation either interested me or confirmed something I believed?

2. List as many experiences where you began noticing things, or conversations about things, that you were planning on purchasing or had already purchased. A great example of this is when you buy a new car and suddenly you see that model of car everywhere when you never noticed them before. There wasn't a sudden increase in these cars on the road; they just seem to start "popping out" at you all of a sudden. This is also an example of the R.A.S. bringing to conscious awareness information that it believes you now consider important.

3. Answer the following questions:

- Do you believe you tend to notice sweet foods or foods that aren't on your diet more so than people who aren't overweight?

- Do these foods and commercials for foods tend to "jump out at you"?

- Based on what you've learned, what role do you believe the R.A.S. plays in you noticing these foods?

Now, before you begin actively changing your negative core beliefs into healthy ones that support you in permanent weight loss, let's learn about one more tool the subconscious uses to sabotage your efforts—the Inner Critic.

SUMMARY

Key Points

- Unlike the Critical Gateway, which is a psychological construct, the R.A.S. is a set of connected nuclei that connects the brain stem with the cortex.

- The R.A.S. has many functions, but the one most relevant to our ability to change core beliefs is that it acts as a filter, determining what information that comes in through our senses is brought to conscious awareness and what is sent directly to the subconscious.

- At any given time, we take in millions of bits of information per second through our senses. This includes incoming sensory information that we see, feel, smell, and taste. Our conscious mind is only able to process 40 bits per second of that information. Our R.A.S. determines, out of all of that information, which 40 bits we become aware of consciously.

- Some great examples of the R.A.S. at work are a mother's ability to become aware of her child crying among dozens of other children making similar noises, and your ability to pick your own name being spoken out of a crowded room of people talking despite your name not being spoken louder than the ambient noise in the room.

- This function of the R.A.S. developed, in part, as a survival mechanism designed to let us know what needs our immediate attention.

- The R.A.S. has a tendency to filter out of conscious awareness things that do not support your existing core beliefs while bringing to your attention those things that do.

- If something in your environment, a conversation in a crowded room for example, contains information that contradicts your existing core beliefs, it's often filtered out by the R.A.S. You won't even notice it. However, if what's being discussed in that conversation confirms your existing beliefs, you will often be able to pick it out among all of the other noise in the room.

- If an experience can't be ignored or filtered out of consciousness, for example, you are having a private conversation with someone when you receive information that directly contradicts your core beliefs, the Critical Gateway will then cause you not to believe it. In this way, the R.A.S. and the Critical Gateway function together to preserve your existing core beliefs.

- Once you reprogram your R.A.S. based on your new core beliefs that support you in losing weight, it will constantly bring to your attention information and experiences that support you in your goals.

What This Has To Do With Weight Loss

Losing weight and keeping it off requires gathering new resources and paying attention to new things. This can be as simple as noticing all of the examples in your life of people who have achieved your same goals, or noticing and becoming aware of all of the experiences of life that reaffirm your self-worth and value. The Reticular Activating System determines what you pay attention to, specifically what is brought to your conscious awareness. Reprogramming the R.A.S. to notice the things that empower you—instead of putting you into an emotional state that leads to unhealthy eating, sadness, or any other thoughts and feelings that lead to weight loss sabotage—is an important part of the permanent weight loss process. The information you learned in this chapter will soon be used to reprogram the Reticular Activating System to work for you to enable you to more easily reach your permanent weight loss goals.

You Are Ready To Move To The Next Chapter When . . .

- You understand that the R.A.S. acts as a filter, determining what you become aware of in situations where there are competing distractions.

- You understand the role the R.A.S. plays in preserving your existing core beliefs by only bringing to your conscious awareness things that reinforce and support those beliefs.

- You begin to understand how and why you tend to notice things that make it hard to stay with your diet.

- You have watched the tutorial video for this chapter and are following the included instructions to actively use your Hypnotherapy Audio Sessions (if you have the full *Fat to Fearless®* program).

- You have completed the exercises for this chapter in the Success Guide and Workbook (if you have the full *Fat to Fearless®* program).

CHAPTER 8

INNER CRITIC

The Inner Critic is the third of the three important tools of the subconscious mind used to keep your existing beliefs from changing.

The Inner Critic is that negative voice inside your head that often keeps you feeling bad about yourself and has far more to do with keeping you overweight than you realize. Have you ever wondered where this voice comes from? If you're like most people you probably assume it's just part of "you." However, it might surprise you to learn that you weren't born saying bad things to yourself and that this negative internal dialogue is actually a learned response that operates subconsciously. Changing this negative inner voice to one that supports you instead of criticizes you is integral to eliminating the compulsion to emotionally eat as well as self-sabotage many other areas of your life. The Inner Critic is also the third mechanism of your subconscious that reinforces, and makes it difficult to change, your negative core beliefs.

The Inner Critic is born out of a child's response to early socialization and what they perceive as the expectation of their tribe. Humans are tribal animals, which helps us understand how the expectations of others impacts us as children as we grow and socialize.

Thousands of years of evolution have hard-wired into our brain that we are dependent on our tribe for survival. If you go back to the dawn of civilization, you will find that individuals needed the tribe functioning together to provide safety from animals, shelter from the elements, and to gather and hunt food. If you were kicked out of your tribe, you would likely die.

Knowing how to behave in order to stay within the safety of the tribe was a matter of life or death. Fitting in was a survival skill and our minds developed ways to ensure we behaved appropriately. This mechanism became our Inner Critic.

When you were born, your world was mostly free of rules. The things you were prohibited from doing were usually related to your safety and survival. As soon as you were old enough to socially interact, things begin to change. It was no longer, *don't put that in your mouth* or *don't stick that in the electrical socket*, but *act like a lady* (or gentleman), *don't be rude, don't cry, you don't want to be fat, be seen and not heard,* and hundreds of other messages, many of them conflicting with each other. It is not only directives on what to do, how to be, and how to act that were relayed to you, but also the ideas about what happens if you don't follow these rules.

You learned that you were a "bad" boy or girl when you didn't live up to these expectations. As you remember from the chapter on how beliefs are formed, it is usually during this time that you adopted your negative core beliefs about yourself. As a child, you did not have the emotional or intellectual maturity to evaluate what you were told. You simply accepted it as true, and without the Critical Gateway to filter these experiences, they became embedded in your subconscious.

But what happened when you were old enough to crawl or toddle away from your parents and interact with the world without them there to tell you if you were being bad or good? After all, this was critical information to have to ensure you didn't do something so grievous that you were "disowned" by your tribe.

What happened was you developed and carried an internalized version of your parents with you to continue to guide you. Your internal dialogue asked what your parents would think in situations where you were uncertain about how to act.

You started this process at an early age, constructing "soundtracks" of what your parents might tell you. Unfortunately, since those soundtracks were designed to keep you in line they were made of memories of times when you were being corrected and therefore they tended to be negative. You replayed those negative soundtracks until they become second nature. You no longer needed someone else to criticize you when you believed you had done wrong because you created an automatic "voice" in your head that did it for you.

This "voice" also strongly affected how you felt because it reinforced the experiences that resulted in your specific negative core beliefs. If you believed you were unlovable, every time you did something wrong this inner critical voice would reaffirm that for you in your own head. As you grew, this process passed from conscious to subconscious and developed into a self-sustaining program in your mind that evolved into the Inner Critic. By the time you become an adult you do not remember a time it wasn't there and think that it's just "you."

If you were raised in a consistently loving and caring environment where your caretakers were very conscious of the long-term effects their interactions with you would have on your long-term emotional health, this inner voice is nurturing and gently nudges you in the right direction. For many, however, this voice ranges from slightly critical to outright abusive.

It's important to understand that the Inner Critic is not necessarily an actual representation of your parents and childhood experiences. Because it originated as an internal check to correct your behavior and is based on times you were corrected or reprimanded, it is usually formed out of the worst ideas you had of your caretakers at an age when you were too young to make such an assessment.

Unfortunately, you can never be "good enough" to satisfy the Inner Critic and the way this negative voice goes about pushing you to "be better" usually ends up making you feel worse about yourself. To make matters worse, you began creating the Inner Critic at such a young age that you can't remember a time when it was not there. You consider that voice to be who you actually are, as opposed to just a program based on your internalized ideas of what is expected of you. By the time you became an adult, you had no recollection of not having this voice inside your head, and it has been influencing your behaviors and your self-esteem ever since.

It is important that you realize that this critical voice is not who you are. It will tell you that you are stupid or a loser or that you are fat, but it is not who you are. It is only a psychological mechanism developed in childhood, and it is based on the worst possible interpretation of what, as a child, you believed was expected of you in order to have "value" and be worthy of love.

This voice was designed to keep you in line with what you believed you needed to do or who you believed you needed to be so that you would fit in with your family and be loved by those you depended on for survival. Whether these expectations were positive or negative is irrelevant.

For example, if you grew up in a family system where your parents were extreme pessimists and cynical about the world, then being upbeat and happy would cause dissonance between you and the family you needed. To ensure that you fit into your family system, your Inner Critic would evolve to become pessimistic and cynical and would criticize you when you were overly optimistic. Although later in life this might keep you from being happy, at the time it served you well and ensured you stayed within the guidelines of the family system.

I think of the Inner Critic as the henchman of your negative core beliefs, constantly telling you things that make you feel bad about yourself. In response to these bad feelings we often end up engaging in behaviors like overeating that reinforce beliefs that do not serve us in reaching our goals and achieving our dreams. This includes your goal of losing weight and keeping it off.

That is why changing this Inner Critic into a loving and supportive voice is key to building and maintaining the new belief systems you will soon develop to lose weight and keep it off. As you will soon learn, another reason for disempowering the Inner Critic is the emotional toll it takes on you and how often it is the source of your desire to emotionally eat to feel better.

Every behavior develops because it served a purpose at one point. When you were young, having a voice in your head that criticized you for doing things that might get you in trouble served a purpose. As an adult, however, this voice is no longer needed to keep you following the rules. You now have an adult mind that is better equipped to make its own decisions about what to believe and what rules to follow. If you need to, you can now create your own tribe and support system around healthier beliefs.

To go from *Fat to Fearless*® your Inner Critic must change to support you in reaching your goals. For the Inner Critic to change, your negative core beliefs must also change because they are the script from which the Inner Critic draws its conclusions about you and how you "measure up."

In the next chapter you will uncover your specific negative core beliefs so you can then begin to change them into beliefs that support you in weight loss and in living the life you want. Before that though, it's important for our future work together that you learn to identify the voice of the Inner Critic in your head and be able to tell it apart from the real you.

Complete the following exercise in your Success Guide and Workbook. If you don't have the full program with the workbook and videos, I would encourage you to invest in yourself by downloading it from www.fattofearless.com. Otherwise, complete the following exercise on your own paper:

EXERCISE: YOUR INNER CRITIC SPEAKS!

For the next week, keep your *Fat to Fearless*® Success Guide and Workbook with you throughout the day and use the appropriate pages to write every thought that enters your mind that you can attribute to the Inner Critic. You will know these thoughts because they are accompanied by negative feelings. Also, anytime the word "should" passes through your mind and is followed by a bad feeling it is almost always the Inner Critic speaking. The word "should" implies an internal judgment that you should be different, or doing something differently, than what you are.

Write what the Inner Critic actually says, instead of writing *about* what it says. For example, you would not write:

"The Inner Critic says bad things to me about me not being good enough and that I'm a loser."

Instead, you would write exactly what it says to you, which may sound like:

"You're such a loser."
"There you go screwing up again."
"You're so fat, you're never going to lose weight."

Further in the program you will begin to understand the power of words. Later, when we disempower this negative voice, it will be important to understand the exact words it uses when it talks to you.

Your goal in this exercise is threefold:

First, understand the very specific language your Inner Critic uses to speak to you.

Second, get some distance from the Inner Critic by identifying that it is separate from the real you.

Third, begin to observe that almost all of your bad feelings, and most of the negative behaviors you want to change (like emotional eating) are caused directly or indirectly by your emotional response to what the Inner Critic says to you.

SUMMARY

Key Points

- The Inner Critic is the negative voice inside your head that you hear every time you criticize yourself for something you did or didn't do or because you are "less than" in any way.

- While you may consider this voice to be "you," in actuality it's an internalized subconscious response from childhood.

- It is important that you realize that this critical voice is not who you are.

- All behavior develops because it at one time served a purpose. Many of our problems in life are the result of behaviors that developed early in childhood, which at the time served a positive purpose. However, these behaviors often cause problems later in our adult lives. The Inner Critic is an example of this.

- Humans are tribal animals. During our early evolution, much of our survival depended upon our ability to fit in with the tribe.

- The Inner Critic developed as a way of self-policing yourself to ensure you were living up to expectations so you didn't alienate your tribe or family.

- Any time you deviate from how you believe you "should" be, you will hear the voice of the Inner Critic. This idea of how you should be comes from your core beliefs about yourself and was formed in childhood.

- The Inner Critic helps preserve our negative subconscious beliefs. It convinces us we aren't good enough by setting a standard we can never live up to. You will soon learn that it takes both our conscious and subconscious minds to defeat and transform our Inner Critic.

- How "negative" the Inner Critic is depends on our childhood experiences. The healthier and more supportive your early childhood environment was, the less harsh your Inner Critic is. The more you were criticized as a child or observed unhealthy ways of relating or learned unhealthy expectations, the more harsh and critical your Inner Critic is.

- No matter how critical your Inner Critic is, by using the tools in the *Fat to Fearless®* program you will be able to transform it into a healthier and more supportive voice.

- It's important to become consciously aware of what the Inner Critic says to you that impacts you in a negative way. We will use this information later to disempower the Inner Critic and change it to a healthier and more supportive voice.

What This Has To Do With Weight Loss

An important concept you will soon learn is that all behaviors are driven by emotional states. Nowhere is this more easily seen than the desire to eat for any reason other than being physically hungry. We reach for food when we feel bad, and more times than not we feel bad as a result of the negative things we say to ourselves. Sometimes we are consciously aware we do this, other times it happens so automatically we don't even realize it. Regardless of how aware we are of what we say to ourselves that puts us in the state that drives us to eat emotionally, the Inner Critic is almost always behind it.

The *Fat to Fearless®* program is about changing your subconscious to ensure you are in the emotional states that drive not just temporary weight loss, but long-term success and happiness with keeping the weight off and feeling good about yourself. To do this, we must change this negative voice in your mind to one that *supports* you instead of making you feel bad. The information you learned in this chapter, especially the exercise where you learn to hear that voice in your mind and understand what it says to you, is used to do that as you continue through the program.

You Are Ready To Move To The Next Chapter When . . .

- You understand that the negative voice in your head that criticizes you isn't actually you but is a "program" you developed in childhood to make sure you are doing what you thought you "should" be doing as well as how you thought you should be.

- You are open to accepting that what this voice says to you, about you, isn't true.

- You understand that the bad feelings that often drive you to eat for reasons other than being hungry come from what the Inner Critic says to you.

- You have developed the ability to become consciously aware of when the Inner Critic is speaking to you and can clearly identify it from your other thoughts.

- You have watched the tutorial video for this chapter and are following the included instructions to actively use your Hypnotherapy Audio Sessions (if you have the full *Fat to Fearless*® program).

- You have completed the exercises for this chapter in the Success Guide and Workbook (if you have the full *Fat to Fearless*® program).

At this point, you've taken in a lot of information. It's important to give yourself time to actually process what you're learning and develop new skills before moving on too quickly. The goal isn't just for you to learn new things consciously, but for you to take the time to allow them to sink in at a deeper level. This chapter is a turning point in that the skill of being able to identify the voice of the Inner Critic is foundational to all of our work going forward. I would suggest taking a full week to do the exercise in this chapter to become very aware of that critical voice in your mind and begin to see it as separate from you instead of actually being "you."

The time that you take now to fully assimilate and apply what you're learning won't slow you down but actually speed up your results with the program. During any periods of time where I suggest you pause in moving forward to fully process and absorb what you're learning, you will continue to use your Hypnotherapy Audio Sessions included in the program, as the instructions that came with the audios suggest.

CHAPTER 9

UNCOVERING CORE BELIEFS

At this point in the program you should have a clear understanding of the role your subconscious core beliefs play in every area of your life. Your subconscious mind essentially operates to ensure that what you believe at the deepest level is what you experience as true in the world.

Despite what you may consciously believe, the results you're getting in all areas of your life are a result of your subconscious acting on behalf of your core beliefs. If you want to experience something new in the world, like losing weight and keeping it off, you must change the core beliefs that have always prevented that outcome in the past.

One of the biggest challenges, not only with changing your beliefs but also in accepting that you have negative beliefs that are interfering with your life, is that we often aren't consciously aware of what they are. At the conscious level it seems absurd that we would actually believe these things about ourselves.

You've learned already that these beliefs are typically formed in childhood, often from experiences that you don't even remember. You've also learned that once core beliefs are formed, the subconscious mechanisms of the Critical Gateway, Reticular Activating System, and the Inner Critic make it hard to change those beliefs without a proven program that creates subconscious change. Fortunately the *Fat to Fearless*® program is exactly that and the first step to changing your existing core beliefs to ones that support you in creating permanent weight loss is figuring out what your existing beliefs are.

In this chapter you begin to actively work on yourself by uncovering the beliefs that have caused you problems throughout your life, including those that have interfered with your ability to lose weight. After going through this process and understanding what your specific negative core beliefs are, you will then be prepared to take responsibility for transforming your life and your body.

This chapter consists mostly of a variety of exercises to help you uncover your negative core beliefs. The first exercise is based on understanding that the subconscious mind takes your core beliefs as an operating system for your life. Your subconscious constructs your life in a way that ensures those beliefs are proven right. Knowing this, one of the easiest ways to uncover your core beliefs is to look at your life, and then reverse engineer backwards to find what beliefs it took to create a life like yours.

One example of this comes from Richard Bandler, the father and co-creator of Neuro-Linguistic Programming (NLP). I was fortunate enough to personally train with Richard and always enjoyed his real-world examples. I will teach you many of the principles he taught me.

My favorite stories were about when he was hired by software companies to determine what the glitch was in their software that they could not uncover or fix on their own. Richard's background as a scientist and a mathematician made him well suited for this job, but it was his skills of human observation and Neuro-linguistic Programming that usually solved the problem.

He talked about how, when beginning a new consulting project, the very first thing he would do was interview the software engineers who developed the software with the bug. This was not unusual, but the questions he asked them were. He did not ask them about the software itself, but instead asked them about their lives. By applying many of the principles I would later learn from him, he was able to understand where the glitches were in their personal lives, and then understand that those same subconscious issues were undoubtedly playing out in the mental processes they used to construct their software.

One designer had a chronic problem of never finishing anything. He would gather all of the information, material, and resources required to move forward in an area of his life, but never seemed to successfully merge these things together and take the next step. From this, Richard knew to look in the part of the software code that was responsible for putting all of the various elements of the program together to produce a coherent whole. In computer language, he looked for the code that compiled everything before running the program. Once he knew where to look, the glitch was easily found and corrected.

Another software engineer had a habit of always starting over in his personal life. He had multiple jobs that were only lateral moves, never upward. The same was true of his relationships. He had multiple marriages that all seemed to begin and end in the same way without learning any lessons. From this, Richard knew that there was something in the code that was creating a feedback loop causing certain functions to repeat themselves. Once he knew what needed to be changed, it was easy to find and correct.

In much the same way as the examples above, your life is essentially a "played out" example of what is going on in your subconscious. By looking at the outcomes you produce in your life, you can get a sense of the subconscious beliefs that are responsible for those outcomes. Like in the examples above, when you know what is causing the problem, it's easy to correct when you have the right tools.

Complete the following exercises in the Success Guide and Workbook. If you don't have the full program with the workbook and videos, you can download it at: www.fattofearless.com

Otherwise, complete the exercise that follows on your own paper.

In this first exercise you look deeply at your own life to determine what core beliefs would create a life like yours.

EXERCISE: MY LIFE STORY

If you have the complete *Fat to Fearless*® program, turn to the appropriate section of your workbook to do these exercises and be sure to watch the video tutorials.

Step 1

In this first exercise you will write your life story. While you don't have to write a novel, you should include your thoughts and feelings about key areas of your life (relationships, health, finance, etc.) as well as the circumstances that led you to your current status in each of those areas. It is important that at this point it not be an objective analysis, but instead a narrative of your thoughts and feelings about yourself and your life. Do not hold back. Do not try to be politically correct or make yourself sound good. Write with the idea that no one will ever read this but you. Be honest.

Include your struggles with weight in this story, but be sure to include other areas of life as well. As you will learn, issues with your body do not take place in a vacuum and are often intertwined with other areas of your life. Changing your life involves changing your emotions. Changing your emotions requires doing the exercises. If you only read this book, but don't do the exercises, you will gain knowledge but not transformation. Do this exercise now before reading any further in the book.

Step 2

Now that you have written your story, it's time for you to "reverse engineer" your life to uncover your core beliefs.

First, determine how many areas of your life are represented in your story. The most common ones are health, finance, relationships, spirituality, career, and our social lives. A page has been provided in the Success Guide and Workbook for each area.

Next, for each area of your life, write a brief synopsis of how you view your life in this area. For example, for the health category your synopsis may be something like, "I've struggled with weight my entire life. I've gone on countless diets and lost weight only to regain it over and over. It seems the harder I try and the more I want it, the more I fail. Because of my weight, I always feel bad about myself, hold myself back from being more outgoing and social, and I'm not living the life I want to live. I hate exercising, and I feel as if everyone is looking at me and laughing at me for being so overweight and going to the gym. I feel as if it's hopeless, and I just need to accept being fat."

If this is your story, don't worry, we'll change it soon.

Step 3

Our core beliefs are acted on by our subconscious as instructions for how to create our life. When you consciously want to be something that you have always struggled to be, such as to be thin when you are overweight, there will be a conflict with your subconscious. While you may consciously want to lose weight, your subconscious will sabotage you because losing weight would not be compatible with your existing core beliefs. We know this because your body is a reflection of your beliefs, and if you've struggled with being overweight most of your life, your current core beliefs can't be ones that support your weight loss goals.

Underneath the synopsis you just wrote on each workbook page for each of the different areas of your life, ask yourself what core beliefs someone would need to have for their subconscious to create that outcome in that area of their life. Write them down in the table provided on each page underneath the synopsis.

Another way of looking at this is, if my subconscious were trying to prove something to me about myself by creating this outcome, what would it be proving? It is important for you to understand that you also have positive core beliefs, not just negative beliefs. But the focus of our work is to transform the negative into the positive, so these exercises focus on uncovering the beliefs that do not serve you in reaching your goals. Do this exercise for each area of life. Below is a list of common negative core beliefs that you can use as a reference. This list is by no means complete, but it is a good starting point.

Common Negative Core Beliefs

- I'm not good enough.
- I'm a loser.
- I'm innately flawed.
- I'm second best.
- I'm ugly.
- I'm stupid.
- I deserve to be alone.
- I'm unsafe.
- I'm unlovable.
- I'm unworthy.
- Money is bad.
- I don't deserve good things.
- I'm always abandoned.
- No one wants me.
- Intimacy is unsafe.
- If you get to know me, you won't like me.
- I have no control.
- I'm wrong.
- I'm insignificant.
- I'm dirty or not pure.

Step 4

Now turn to the "The Beliefs I'm Changing" page in your Success Guide and Workbook and list the negative core beliefs you have identified from all areas of your life on this one page. If you don't yet have the full program, use your own paper.

Step 5

Now it is time to determine the degree of consciousness you have around these negative core beliefs. This will tell you the degree to which your conscious and subconscious are in conflict about them.

Next to each negative core belief, write a number in the appropriate blank on your "The Beliefs I'm Changing" workbook page that indicates on a scale of 1 to 10 how much you consciously believe or are aware you have this belief, with 1 being *not at all* and 10 being *I am fully aware that I believe this about myself at a core level.*

Now you have a working list of the potential negative core beliefs that may be operating in your life that cause you to self-sabotage yourself, including your ability to lose weight and keep it off. In the next exercise you will refine this list further.

These exercises may at times feel a little overwhelming. I highly encourage you to watch the tutorial videos for each exercise. In these videos I explain the exercise in more detail as well as give additional insights.

EXERCISE: STEM SENTENCES

For all of the exercises in this chapter on uncovering core beliefs, I highly recommend making sure you watch the associated video tutorials. These exercises can seem more complicated than they are in written form but are much more easily understood when explained and demonstrated on video.

This exercise uses stem sentences (I provide the beginning and you fill in the rest) to further uncover your existing core beliefs. The idea behind stem sentences is that if the sentence is structured in a particular way and you complete the sentence without thinking about the answer first, you are more likely to give an answer that comes from the subconscious before editing it with your conscious mind. I often use this technique in sessions to get a better understanding of a client's core beliefs around a particular symptom. *I can't emphasize enough that the answer is the first impulse, thought, or feeling you have.* Our goal is to find out what is in your subconscious. When you take time to think about it, you use the conscious mind and contaminate the answer. Remember you are the only one who will see this, so don't hold back and "edit" your answers.

Step 1

Turn to the Stem Sentences exercise in your Success Guide and Workbook and complete the following sentences with your first impulse, thought, and/or feeling.

1. Relationships are...
   (An example might be "Relationships are hard")

2. Love is...

3. Money is...

4. I'm most afraid of...

5. My body is...

6. Losing weight is...

7. Meeting new people is...

8. I'm secretly afraid people will find out I am...

9. Sex is...

10. Beautiful people are..

11. People think I am...

12. I can't do what I most want because...

13. I'm not someone who can...

14. Fat people are...

15. Thin people are...

You should now have a list of answers to the above questions that came directly from your initial gut response without having thought about them, judged them, or debated them with yourself.

Step 2

Take the list of completed sentences and put them in the appropriate column in your Success Guide and Workbook.

Now add "because I believe I am..." to the end of each sentence above and complete the new sentence with the first unedited response that comes to mind. Your response doesn't have to make sense to your conscious mind. List your responses in the appropriate blank in your Success Guide and Workbook.

Example:

Stem sentence: I'm most afraid of...

Answer to above stem sentence: meeting new people

New Stem Sentence: I'm most afraid of meeting new people because I believe I am...

Immediate response that comes to mind: ...Not Good Enough

Do this exercise now for all of the above feelings on your list and write the answers in your Success Guide and Workbook or on your own paper.

Step 3

Take your list of responses to the "I am" stem sentences that are negative and add them to the "The Beliefs I'm Changing" page in your workbook. For any beliefs that are duplicates of the ones you uncovered in previous exercises, put another mark in the "# of times occurred" column so you know this core belief has shown up more than once now. For any new beliefs that were uncovered that you added to the list, just like in the previous exercise, be sure to rate on a scale of 1 to 10 the degree to which you believe or are aware that this is true about you.

At the completion of this exercise, you should begin to have a sense of what negative core beliefs are subconsciously operating in your life that may be sabotaging you in various ways, including weight loss. In the next exercise, you will begin to understand what negative core beliefs may specifically be connected to your weight issues.

EXERCISE: SYMPTOM CYCLE BELIEFS

For all of the exercises in this chapter on uncovering core beliefs, I highly recommend making sure you watch the associated video tutorials. These exercises can seem more complicated than they are in written form, but are much more easily understood when explained and demonstrated on video.

Step 1

In this exercise, you will go back to the previous exercise "The Symptom Cycle" and find the negative word that you determined you call yourself in the moments you feel worst about your body and the list of emotions you created when you completed the sentence: Being *(insert the word you call yourself)* makes me feel so _____.

Rewrite the list of emotions from the previous exercise in the appropriate blanks in your workbook.

Step 2

Now, inserting the negative word you use to refer to yourself and one of the feelings from the list, complete the following sentence with the first thing that comes to your mind without thinking about it:

Being *(insert your word: fat, etc.)* makes me feel so *(insert one emotion from your list: angry, sad, etc.)* because I secretly believe I am _____.

Add your answer to your "The Beliefs I'm Changing" workbook page.

Step 3

Repeat this with each of the emotions on your list. Take your list of responses to these "I am..." stem sentences and add each of them to the "The Beliefs I'm Changing" page in your workbook. Any beliefs that are duplicates of the ones you uncovered in previous exercises, put another mark in the "#" of times occurred column so you know this core belief has shown up again. For any new beliefs that were uncovered that you added to the list, just like in the previous exercise, be sure to rate on a scale of 1 to 10 the degree to which you believe or are aware that this is true about you.

EXERCISE: REFINING THE LIST

Now that you have what is a fairly substantial list on your "The Beliefs I'm Changing" workbook page, it is time for us to refine it down to the top 5 that you are going to focus on transforming into healthier positive beliefs.

Step 1

The first step in refining your list is to make sure that everything you have listed is an actual belief. Sometimes when completing the stem sentences you may list an emotion instead of a belief. Take the following stem sentence for example:

"Being fat makes me feel so angry because I am sad."

Assuming "fat" is the word you call yourself in your worst moments and the emotion was "angry." In this instance, instead of completing the sentence with a belief, the emotion "sad" was used.

Sometimes it may not be easy to tell the difference between an emotion and a belief. As a general rule, beliefs tend to be constant and not changing and emotions tend to be more malleable based on circumstances.

For example, if one of your core beliefs is "I'm not good enough" then that belief, at a deep level, is with you all the time. This doesn't mean that you are always actively thinking this in every moment, but it means regardless of what is going on externally, if you go deep within yourself you'll find that you believe this about yourself at a core level *most of the time.* In this example, external circumstances and personal achievements may cause you to feel better about yourself for a while, but you eventually return to your core belief of being not good enough.

Feelings on the other hand tend to come and go and rise and decrease significantly based on what is going on in the moment. Often, you are aware of negative emotions more strongly and acutely than you are your negative core beliefs.

For example, you may feel strong sadness that you can't get off your mind and that dominates your emotional landscape because of an event or situation. However, you typically don't walk around all day with the negative core belief "I'm unlovable" stuck on repeat in your head. At least not consciously.

Feelings tend to be the conscious manifestation of our subconscious beliefs, which makes it easy to understand why our first response to "I am" stem sentence questions designed to find beliefs are often emotions instead.

Go through your list of potential core beliefs on your "The Beliefs I'm Changing" page and eliminate emotions. Below is a list of common emotions. While technically, all of these aren't emotions, they are common responses to the stem sentences related to being overweight that should be eliminated as beliefs. This list is by no means comprehensive but can act as a guide.

If these are on your list, put a mark through them.

Common Emotions

- Sad
- Happy/Joyful
- Angry
- Afraid
- Optimistic

- Anxious (Anxiety is actually a fear of feeling specific emotions, yet it can still be considered an emotion on its own for our purposes.)
- Embarrassed
- Surprised
- Unsatisfied
- Lonely
- Regretful
- Overwhelmed
- Bored
- Ashamed
- Guilty

Note: When Words Can Be Both Emotions and Beliefs There are certain words that seem as if they could be both a belief and an emotion and don't easily fall into one camp or the other. Guilt, lonely, and angry are great examples. Allow me to illustrate the subtle differences:

If I am *feeling angry* (emotion), it is certainly an emotion, yet it does not necessarily mean *I am an angry person* (belief).

Likewise, *feeling lonely* isn't the same as the belief *I am alone*.

As a rule of thumb, for these few words that define states that aren't so easily put in a feeling/belief category, use the following to help you decide if it's a feeling or a belief.

A. If you are aware that this is something you feel only in certain situations and it doesn't pervade your life, it is most likely a feeling.

B. Take the word and put it into the following sentence and see if it feels true: "I am a *(insert word)* person."

If "guilty" were the word, then the sentence would be "I am a guilty person." If you have an immediate reaction that feels as if that's not true, then it is probably an emotion you are feeling because of experiences filtered through core beliefs and not the belief itself.

Lastly, when doing this check there is a difference between an immediate inner reaction of feeling as if "that's not true" and a conflicted reaction of denying it because you don't want it to be true. If you find internal conflict when doing the exercise, more deep searching may be necessary.

Step 2

Now, looking at the list that remains, choose the top four core beliefs that you want to change. These should be the ones that you feel create the most challenge for you and, based on what you've learned so far, are causing you to self-sabotage your weight loss efforts. If being "not good enough," "unlovable," or any shade of these beliefs are on your list, then I would definitely suggest choosing these as part of the four.

Step 3

After you've chosen the four beliefs you want to change, look at the number you assigned each belief in the prior exercises to indicate how conscious you are that this belief is operating in your life. If all of the four beliefs you've chosen are ones that you have a high degree of awareness in, meaning you already know or believe they are there, then choose a fifth belief to add to the list that you ranked as you being less consciously aware of. If your list of four is already varied, choose a fifth to add to the list that you would also like to change.

Often, beliefs that we are less conscious of, and resist acknowledging, serve as linch pins holding together the structure of some of the other negative core beliefs.

You should now have a list of five negative core beliefs that you are now going to begin actively changing into core beliefs that are healthier and more positive and that will support you in losing weight and keeping it off.

SUMMARY

Key Points

- An important step in changing your core beliefs is knowing what they are.

- These exercises are designed to help you uncover your core beliefs and are best performed without "thinking about them" or editing your responses. This helps ensure the answers come from the subconscious mind without interference from the conscious mind.

- One of the best ways of determining what your core beliefs are is to examine your life with the understanding that your subconscious has constructed it from your core beliefs.

- The effects of core beliefs in your life are rarely confined to just one area. Looking for evidence of themes throughout multiple areas of your life can also help you identify subconscious core beliefs you may not be aware of.

- The more times you see a potential core belief operating in multiple areas of your life, the more certain you can be that it is actually one of your core beliefs.

- One way of eliciting core beliefs from your subconscious is by using stem sentences. Stem sentences are a technique in which you are given the first part of the sentence that has been designed to produce a subconscious response when automatically completing the sentence without thinking about the response first.

- If at any time you feel overwhelmed or aren't completely clear on how to do an exercise, be sure to watch the tutorial video on the exercise.

What This Has To Do With Weight Loss

If you've suffered from life-long weight issues caused by emotional eating and self-sabotage, your subconscious core beliefs about yourself and what you deserve are most definitely part of the problem. Before you can begin to change those beliefs into healthier ones that support you in permanent weight loss, you must first uncover what they are.

You Are Ready To Move To The Next Chapter When . . .

- You have watched the tutorial video for this chapter and are following the included instructions to actively use your Hypnotherapy Audio Sessions (if you have the full *Fat to Fearless®* program).

- You have completed the exercises for this chapter in the Success Guide and Workbook (if you have the full *Fat to Fearless®* program).

- You have determined five core beliefs you presently have that you will change into new and more positive beliefs to support you in transforming your body and reaching your weight loss goals.

PART IV

NEW BODY BELIEFS

CHAPTER 10

CHANGING YOUR BELIEFS

In Part IV, you take the next step on your *Fat to Fearless®* journey and transform your negative core beliefs into positive ones that support you in your weight loss goals.

At this point you know how core beliefs are formed and maintained in your mind and why they are so difficult to change without a program designed to work at the subconscious level. You also have a good idea of what your own negative core beliefs are that are contributing, if not completely causing, your weight issues. You also have a good understanding of the Symptom Cycle, which says that the way we feel about being overweight is the emotional cause of the behaviors that keep us overweight, and the role it plays in causing weight loss failure. You are now ready to look beyond the symptom of being overweight and begin working on the root cause, your negative core beliefs.

In therapy, there is one fundamental question that I know will determine whether or not a person will follow through, do the work it takes to succeed, and complete therapy with the positive results they consciously say that they want. That question is this: *Have you suffered enough?*

More than anything else, the answer to this question determines your success. In my private practice, I rarely accept clients in their 20s because they usually have not suffered enough to truly be ready to change. They have not run the same old patterns long enough and produced the same ineffective results enough times for them to accept that they cannot continue doing and thinking as they always have and get a different result.

There are of course exceptions to this with young clients, but most people need to have lived long enough to have tried enough of the same patterns to reach the inescapable conclusion that something at a fundamental level must change. **For that to happen, the suffering caused by doing things the same way has to be greater than the fear of changing.**

The very first thing you must do to begin changing your core beliefs is consciously ask yourself if you have suffered enough that you are willing to do things differently. Are you ready to let go of quick fixes and diet scams and do the deep, inner work that on some level you have always suspected needed to be done to heal yourself? Are you finally ready to persevere through what may be the most difficult task of your life because you know, while it may not be easy, that it will be worth it? Are you ready to lose weight by gaining life? If yes, then you are ready to begin this work.

If your conscious answer to having suffered enough is "yes," then use the "Have I Suffered Enough?" Hypnotherapy Audio Session, included with the full program, to go within and ask your subconscious if this is true at the subconscious level and if it is ready to support you in making this change.

The next step in this process is to understand specifically what you must do to change your existing core beliefs. You already know more than you realize about this process from what you've already learned. Remember that your existing core beliefs are maintained by:

The Critical Gateway, which acts as a barrier between the conscious and subconscious and filters out any experiences that contradict your existing core beliefs.

The Reticular Activating System (R.A.S.) is a part of the brain that is responsible for determining what, out of all of the information coming in through our senses, we become consciously aware of. It determines what we pay attention to and is programmed to focus on what confirms our existing beliefs. Because of the R.A.S., we are always aware of experiences and information that confirms what we already believe while frequently never noticing contradictory information.

Your Inner Critic is the negative voice in your head that criticizes you and makes you feel bad. Subsequently you then self-soothe with food (or just feel too demotivated to exercise, etc.), which in turn just reinforces your negative core beliefs about who you are and what you deserve.

Now that you understand that these three mechanisms of the subconscious mind conspire to keep your existing beliefs in place, it makes sense that to change your core beliefs you must bypass the critical factor to reach your subconscious mind, reprogram your R.A.S. to search for evidence that confirms your new healthier beliefs instead of the old ones that kept you overweight, as well as transform the Inner Critic so that this internal voice doesn't put you in an emotional place that recreates the Symptom Cycle that we discussed and causes you to reach out for food to feel better.

Let's begin transforming your negative core beliefs now! To change your negative core beliefs into positive ones you must:

1. Bypass the Critical Gateway so that the new beliefs you are wanting to program in can reach your subconscious.

2. Reprogram your Reticular Activating System (R.A.S.) to search for evidence in your environment in a way that will provide constant conscious reinforcement of your new beliefs.

3. Disempower your Inner Critic so that it is no longer creating emotional states that drive behaviors that feed into the old negative core beliefs you are working to change.

I have devoted a chapter to each of these three tasks with exercises and tools to allow you to accomplish these three things and produce powrful change.

Before we launch into changing your negative core beliefs, the first step is deciding what new beliefs you want to replace them with. Well-formed, healthy core beliefs are:

1. Life-Affirming—They expand possibilities and aware-ness, and allow for you to continuously unfold your potential in positive ways.

2. Self-Realized—They are developed within you as a result of life processes that have caused you to decide what you want for your life. They are not introjected, mean-ing someone else's values (like a parent's or peer group's values) forced upon you that you eventually accepted as your own.

3. Independent of Others—Healthy beliefs don't place your value in the hands of others, they operate independ-ent of anyone else. ("People always like me" wouldn't be a healthy core belief because you can't control oth-ers. However, "I am likable" would be healthy because it places the power to determine how you "are" within your own hands regardless of other people.)

While we want our positive core beliefs to be stated in the positive, meaning what we want and not what we don't want, sometimes knowing what we don't want is a great place to start. The following exercise will take you through the process of deciding what new beliefs you are going to be creating for yourself.

EXERCISE: MY NEW BELIEFS

If you have the *Fat to Fearless*® Success Guide and Workbook, turn to the appropriate section and do this exercise now. Also, be sure to watch the instructional video related to this exercise.

For those of you who only have the book and not the full program, instructions for the exercise are below:

1. Go back to your list of uncovered negative core beliefs on your "The Beliefs I'm Changing" workbook page. On your "My New Core Beliefs" workbook page, or on your own paper, transfer over your top five negative core beliefs that you want to change.

2. In the column next to the negative core beliefs, write a corresponding positive belief next to each negative core belief. This will give you a second column of things you would like to believe about yourself right next to the old negative beliefs you're going to begin changing.

   It's important that these new beliefs be phrased in the positive, how you want to be and not how you don't want to be. For example, if one of your negative core beliefs is that you're "a loser", you wouldn't want the positive belief to be "not a loser." Your positive core belief in this example may be something like "I'm a winner" or "I'm more than good enough," etc.

3. Write down your top five life goals that you want to accomplish over the next three years. Make sure one of these goals is something you plan to do in the next six months. Losing a specific amount of weight in this time frame may be this goal!

4. Determine if the new beliefs you listed in step 2 empower you to achieve the goals you just listed. Ask yourself, "If I had these core beliefs would it make it easier or harder to reach these goals?" Also, determine if any of these beliefs are in conflict with your goals. If they are, either the goal or the core belief must change.

   For example, if one of the negative core beliefs you want to replace is "people don't like me and I'm better off being alone" and the new positive core belief you want to adopt is "I am likable and a sociable and outgoing person," but one of your goals is to take a job at a single-manned Antarctic research station, your goal and desired core belief are in conflict.

5. If you have struggled with weight your entire life, I suggest also including the following beliefs if they are not already on your list:

I am lovable.

I am worthy.

I am more than good enough.

I deserve to be thin (or descriptive word of your choice) *and happy!*

Now that you have decided on the new positive beliefs to replace your existing negative beliefs, let's get started doing exactly that.

SUMMARY

Key Points

- At this point you understand how core beliefs are formed in childhood. You also understand the mechanisms of the mind that make it difficult to change your core beliefs on your own without techniques to reach the subconscious. You also have a good idea of what some of your negative core beliefs are as well as how they have contributed to your inability to lose weight.

- The fundamental question that will determine if you will follow through and do the subconscious work of changing your mind and body is: *Have you suffered enough?*

- You have suffered enough when the pain of doing things the way you always have and getting the results you've always gotten is greater than your conscious and subconscious fear of change.

- The first step in determining if you have suffered enough is to have an honest conversation with yourself. If your conscious answer is "yes," then use the "Have I Suffered Enough?" Hypnotherapy Audio Session to go within and ask your subconscious: *Am I ready to let go of quick fixes and diet scams and do the deep, inner work that on some level I have always suspected needed to be done to heal myself and my heart?* If your conscious and subconscious answer is "yes," then you are ready to move forward with changing your core beliefs.

- To change your core beliefs you must:

  1. Bypass the critical factor so that your new beliefs reach the subconscious.

2. Reprogram your R.A.S. to constantly bring to your awareness evidence that your new positive beliefs are true.

3. Change the Inner Critic so that it no longer makes you feel bad about yourself and reinforces your negative self-views.

- You must decide what new, healthier beliefs you want to install in your subconscious so that you can use the *Fat to Fearless*® program to create those changes.

- Healthy beliefs are life-affirming, self-realized, and independent of others.

What This Has To Do With Weight Loss

Everything you have learned so far has been building up to changing your core beliefs to give your subconscious mind a new blueprint for your life that will support you in reaching and maintaining your weight loss goals. This chapter summarizes much of what you've learned so far and prepares you to begin the actual work of changing your negative core beliefs into positive ones.

You Are Ready To Move To The Next Chapter When . . .

- You have created your list of five new positive core beliefs to replace your existing negative ones.

- You have watched the tutorial video for this chapter (if you have the full *Fat to Fearless*® program).

- You have completed the exercises for this chapter in the Success Guide and Workbook (if you have the full *Fat to Fearless*® program).

CHAPTER 11

BYPASSING THE CRITICAL GATEWAY

N ow that you know what new beliefs you want, we can begin changing your old negative beliefs to the new positive ones that will help you reach your weight loss goals. To transform subconscious beliefs you must bypass the Critical Gateway, reprogram your R.A.S., and disempower the Inner Critic. In this chapter you will learn to bypass the Critical Gateway to allow new ideas, specifically the new positive core beliefs, to reach the subconscious. There are five primary ways of bypassing the Critical Gateway.

1. **Repetition.** When presented with a new idea often enough, it eventually works its way through the Critical Gateway. As you wear down the Critical Gateway, it begins to accept the information as true, and it then allows the new information into the subconscious. An example of this is when a person believes they feel fine, but if enough people tell them they look sick throughout the day they will soon start feeling that way.

   Repetition is one of the keys to the entire *Fat to Fearless*® program. If you stay on course—and diligently do all of the exercises—new ideas, beliefs, and programming will eventually reach your subconscious and make lasting change.

2. **Emotional Experiences.** When you are in a highly emotional state the Critical Gateway moves aside, and your subconscious is open to information and suggestion. The subconscious is also known as the emotional mind. This is why a single traumatic event can have a huge impact on you for years or even a lifetime. Impacting the subconscious is a combination of repetition and emotion. The more emotion that is involved, the less repetition that is needed to create change.

3. **Activating Survival Mechanisms.** Any time you are startled or in fear, the Critical Gateway moves aside and your subconscious is open. This function of the Critical Gateway, like much of what you are learning about the subconscious, developed as a survival mechanism. Several thousand years ago if a neighboring tribe suddenly came over the hills running toward your village with clubs in hand, there was no time for debate. In these emergencies the best way of ensuring survival was for the conscious-critical-thinking mind to move aside and turn to the leader for instructions, which would go straight into the subconscious and be acted upon by the group.

This is why hypnotherapists often shock or surprise their clients by raising their voice in the middle of inducing hypnosis. This activates the client's startle response so the hypnotherapists next command—which is usually to go deeper into hypnosis—will immediately be acted upon by the subconscious. In hypnotherapy this is called Rapid or Shock Inductions.

4. **Overwhelm or Overload.** The Critical Gateway exists partially in the conscious mind and partially in the subconscious mind. The parts that exist in the subconscious are comprised of the belief-based filters originating from

subconscious beliefs of which we have absolutely no awareness, and meta-programs that are subconscious preferences for how we filter information that is not necessarily related to our core beliefs.

An example of a meta-program would be, if you were to look at five objects on a table, would you first notice the ways they are similar or the ways they are different? This is a meta-program that defines whether or not you sort-for-sameness or sort-for-difference. There are dozens of meta-programs like this that influence how you perceive, process, and sort incoming information. Everyone has a different combination of master meta-programs that they predominantly use in most circumstances, as well as meta-programs that they use contextually in different circumstances.

While meta-programs can be useful to understand, it is the part of the Critical Gateway that is contained in the conscious mind that is mostly responsible for rejecting information that is not compatible with our existing beliefs. For this reason, bypassing the Critical Gateway is mostly about bypassing the judgments of the conscious mind.

One of the best ways to do this is by overloading or overwhelming it. Remember the conscious mind only has a fraction of the processing ability of your subconscious. Studies show the conscious mind can only hold and process about seven things (plus or minus 2) at any given time. Anything beyond that goes into the subconscious.

Your *Fat to Fearless*® Hypnotherapy Audio Sessions use overwhelm by presenting multiple overlaid audio tracks, each with different suggestions, to overwhelm the conscious mind and bypass the Critical Gateway to reach the subconscious. Anytime you feel overloaded or overwhelmed, your subconscious is more open to being influenced.

5. **Operating Outside of Conscious Awareness.** Since the area of the Critical Gateway that we want to bypass is in the conscious mind, it makes sense that if information is never even perceived by the conscious mind, this part of the Critical Gateway would also be bypassed. There are a variety of ways of doing this.

In conversational hypnotherapy, key words and phrases are often covertly embedded, through pauses and tonal voice shifts, in what appears to be a normal conversation. This is done in a way such that the client never consciously perceives what the therapist is doing. Subsequently, the part of the Critical Gateway located in the conscious mind never has a chance to object to the information the hypnotherapist is imbedding in the client's subconscious.

Technology is another great way of doing this. Subliminal software flashes messages on your computer screen that are too fast for you to consciously read or perceive but are easily perceived by the subconscious. If you have the full *Fat to Fearless®* program, you have access to my subliminal software that's designed to do exactly that. If you don't have the software, you can get it at www.asherfoxweightloss.com/software

All of the activities, exercises, and technologies you are about to use to bypass the Critical Gateway and begin changing your core beliefs will use some combination of these five ways of bypassing the Critical Gateway. The one element that is always used is repetition because it is the most reliable and the easiest one to use to ensure results. In other words, if you do the exercises and listen to your Hypnotherapy Audio Sessions often enough, you will experience change.

Several years ago, NASA did a study designed to gauge the reaction of astronauts to stress and disorientation. They gave each astronaut a pair of specially designed goggles to wear 24 hours a day that altered their vision so that they saw everything upside down. They even slept in these goggles.

At first they were extremely disoriented and experienced all of the signs of stress you would expect to be related to their world being turned 180° upside down 24 hours a day. But an amazing thing happened in the fourth week. One of the astronauts began seeing the world right side up again even though he was still wearing the goggles. Within a matter of days, all of the astronauts' vision reoriented to be being perceived as right side up as well. Over the course of the four weeks that it took for this to happen, their brains had been creating new neural pathways to restructure itself in a way that allowed the astronauts to see normally.

If the subconscious is presented with enough repeated information, it will eventually accept this as its new reality and begin changing the very neural structure of your brain to support this reality. These astronauts were receiving new information 24 hours a day through their goggles that the subconscious eventually responded to by triggering the adaptation necessary for them to function normally in spite of their altered vision.

If you listen to your *Fat to Fearless*® Hypnotherapy Audio Sessions every day, you can't help but experience change because that is the way your mind works.

However, if your expectation is that you will see immediate change and you quit too soon, you will deprive yourself of the real benefit of the *Fat to Fearless*® program—the rewiring of your brain for weight loss success and success in all areas of life.

Look at it this way, if you have been overweight for years and all of the quick fix approaches have not brought you success, isn't it worth taking the chance to devote a few months to transform your body and your life permanently?

Let's begin the process of doing exactly that by using the following tools and exercises to open the Critical Gateway and allow your new beliefs to reach your subconscious.

SUMMARY

Key Points

- To transform old negative core beliefs into new ones, you must bypass the Critical Gateway, reprogram your R.A.S., and disempower the Inner Critic.

- There are five primary ways to bypass the Critical Gateway:

    1. Repetition

    2. Emotional Experiences

    3. Activating Survival Mechanisms

    4. Overwhelm or Overload

    5. Operating Outside of Conscious Awareness

- Repetition is the one element that is always used and combined with the others because it is the most reliable and easiest to use. If exposed to new stimuli long enough, your brain must adapt to this new information.

What This Has To Do With Weight Loss

In the upcoming chapters, you will learn how to bypass the Critical Gateway to adopt new core beliefs that will support reaching your weight loss goals. Your Critical Gateway must be bypassed in order to keep it from rejecting your new beliefs in favor of ones that support your past experience of being unable to achieve permanent weight loss.

You Are Ready To Move To The Next Chapter When . . .

- You have watched the tutorial video for this chapter (if you have the full *Fat to Fearless*® program).

CHAPTER 12

BYPASSING THE CRITICAL GATEWAY
WITH HYPNOTHERAPY

Opening The Critical Gateway:
Hypnotherapy

O ne of the most powerful ways to bypass the Critical
Gateway is Clinical Hypnotherapy. Unfortunately, what
comes to mind when most people hear the word hypnosis
has little to do with what it actually is and how it really works.
Hypnosis is frequently portrayed in the media, television, and
movies as a plot device where people are being controlled
against their will and have little to no idea what they're doing.
In reality, hypnosis is anything but that. Let's dispel some common myths around what is one of the oldest and most powerful
ways to reach the subconscious and heal the mind.

Hypnosis is a natural, yet altered state of mind where the
Critical Gateway is bypassed and there is access to the subconscious mind. Notice I said it was a natural state. While you may
not realize it or call it hypnosis, you actually are going into the
hypnotic state several times a day. A classic example is when
your mind is occupied with other thoughts (overwhelmed/over-
loaded) and you find that you have driven somewhere without

any recollection of the drive. You were in a hypnotic state where your subconscious took over and did the driving for you.

Another common example is watching a movie. To enjoy a movie you must let it bypass your Critical Gateway, otherwise you would constantly be aware that these were actors playing roles with cameras all around them and none of the events on screen were actually taking place. If we didn't suspend our critical thinking while watching, we would rarely be emotionally affected by movies in the way we so often are.

Hypnosis is a natural state that you frequently experience that you can take advantage of to create positive change.

My favorite definition of hypnosis comes from Milton Erickson, one of the most renowned hypnotherapists that ever lived, and whose work transformed the field. Erickson said that hypnosis was simply a state of learning. That has always resonated with me because any time I have used hypnosis with a client it has been to help them learn new behaviors and new ways of being.

Entering into the hypnotic state and gaining access to the virtually unlimited resources of your subconscious mind allows you to take your experiences and use them to create new understandings. This is what learning actually is.

Let's look now at some frequent myths about hypnosis and dispel these misperceptions.

Hypnosis is mind control. A person who is hypnotized is always consciously consenting to what is happening. The dual nature of the mind is that as long as you are awake, the conscious and the subconscious minds are both present to some degree. You are always aware of what is going on when you are in hypnosis, and any time that you object to what's happening, you can make a conscious choice to reject the suggestions being given and even open your eyes and come out of hypnosis altogether. While in hypnosis you can never be forced to go against your moral beliefs.

One of the questions I frequently get asked most is about stage hypnosis and how it works. The most important part of stage hypnosis is selecting the right subject. If you've ever been to a stage hypnosis show, the hypnotist frequently does a series of tests with the audience during which he is carefully looking for the people that are the most responsive or "open to suggestion."

The hypnotist selects a subject that passed the tests that indicate that they either consciously or subconsciously want to participate and want to have the experience of being hypnotized on stage. If any of these participants were given a suggestion that contradicted any of their moral beliefs or something they truly didn't want to do, their conscious mind would take control and not follow through. This is why stage hypnosis subjects are usually given fairly benign instructions, such as the typical "bark like a dog." Very few people have a strong and deep moral opposition to barking like a dog. They may have an opposition to doing something embarrassing, but the stage hypnotist would have weeded out those people in his tests beforehand.

One of the best ways of illustrating this is through a personal example. My first experience with hypnosis was when I was 13 years old and went to a speech therapist to correct a speech impediment. This speech pathologist was also a hypnotherapist that used hypnosis to significantly speed up the process of overcoming speech disorders. During our first session he did what's called Wolberg Arm Levitation. This is a diagnostic test that is often used to determine how deeply someone is in hypnosis. During the procedure the hypnotherapist gives instructions for the subconscious mind to cause the client's arm to begin floating up on its own.

The way I described it to my friends afterwards is the best and simplest explanation to dispel the myth of hypnosis being mind control. I told them, "It was the strangest thing. My arm was floating up all on its very own, I wasn't doing it, but I knew at any time if I wanted to I could have stopped it."

Hypnosis is like sleep. When you watch people who are in hypnosis on television, it often appears as if they are unconscious or not aware of what is going on. This is absolutely not true for most types of hypnosis. The dual nature of the mind is such that the conscious mind is always going to be present to some degree unless you are actually asleep. While those people may be extremely relaxed and have some of the physical signs of sleep, they are actually very aware of what is going on. In fact, hypnosis is often a state of hyper awareness, it is just that that your awareness is focused and turned inward for the purpose of resolving whatever issues you may be seeking hypnosis for. How deeply you are in hypnosis also has little to do with how relaxed you are. Depth of hypnosis is measured by responsiveness to suggestion, not relaxation. In many hypnotherapeutic procedures you may not feel relaxed at all, but still be deeply in hypnosis.

Not everyone can be hypnotized. This is a common misperception created through many hypnotists and hypnotherapists having inadequate training. Unfortunately, hypnotherapy is often unregulated to such a degree that many people can take short courses online and call themselves professional hypnotists and sometimes even hypnotherapists (depending on the state). These people are usually trained in a limited number of styles and techniques and unless someone happens to be a good match for what they learned and is responsive to the specific techniques they were taught, that person often won't go into hypnosis. This has resulted in many people seeing hypnotists and hypnotherapists only to believe they were never hypnotized. The number of hypnotherapists with extensive professional-level training is a very small percentage of those practicing.

The truth is that everyone who sees a hypnotherapist, or begins a program like the *Fat to Fearless*® Hypnotherapy Audio Sessions, has a certain amount of natural responsiveness to suggestion that will increase as they go through the process. It is like athleticism. Everyone has a certain natural level of athleticism that can be improved by practice. Hypnosis works the same way. Hypnosis is actually a learned skill at both the conscious and subconscious levels. Every time you go into hypnosis you develop the ability to go in faster and deeper the next time.

Your initial responsiveness is determined by your past programming and experiences and how guarded you are about expressing your emotions. In hypnosis, your intellectual mind can often work against you. The degree to which you try to analyze what the hypnotherapist is saying or try to "figure it all out" is the degree to which you do not let go. If you are highly analytical, the process can take a little longer, but eventually you become tired of analyzing and let the process happen. Anyone can be hypnotized who is willing to commit to the process and has a well trained and experienced hypnotherapist.

Hypnosis is a single session cure. This myth is also created by poorly trained hypnotherapists who advertise one-session cures, usually with a low long-term success rate. While there are certain conditions that can be cured in one or two sessions, multiple sessions are typically necessary to avoid reoccurrence when dealing with lifelong issues. Also, many hypnotherapists are only trained to work directly with the symptom and not the root cause. This approach almost always leads to an eventual relapse of the problem. This is why the *Fat to Fearless®* program has several different Hypnotherapy Audio Sessions that work to heal and transform both the symptoms and the underlying causes of weight loss failure to enable you to permanently lose weight and keep it off.

You must be in deep hypnosis to get results. Most hypnotherapy is done in a light to medium level of hypnosis. This is because you are given instructions of things to do, visualize, or feel during the session and in the deeper levels of hypnosis you would be so relaxed that you would not want to follow the suggestions. Again, it is mostly for pain management or anesthesia that a hypnotherapist takes a client to deep levels of trance.

You can get stuck in hypnosis. This is not true at all. Certain types of hypnotherapy, such as for pain management or hypnotic anesthesia for surgery, require deep levels of trance. The person may be so relaxed and feel so good that *they don't want to come out of hypnosis*, and choose to reject the hypnotherapist's suggestion to do so (because the client always has control- remember!). But they always have the ability to return to their regular waking consciousness if they choose. In these instances, however, as soon as the person actually falls asleep they will wake up again as they normally would.

Religion is against hypnosis. Hypnosis is a natural mental state endorsed by multiple major medical institutions and associations as a valid healing approach that has nothing to do with religious beliefs. Even the Vatican has said that hypnosis is not a violation of any doctrine. This myth stems from the previously mentioned myth that hypnosis is like mind control.

You must have a weak mind to go into hypnosis. Actually, the opposite of this myth is often true. Hypnosis can't make you do anything against your will. You must not only consciously choose to participate but also use your imagination and follow instructions. The more feeble-minded a person is, the more likely that they will not make the best hypnotic subject.

Hypnosis doesn't work. This myth is predominantly perpetuated by two things. The first is people mystifying hypnosis, and then define "it working" based on the wrong criteria. Essentially, because of modern myth, most people see hypnosis as taking control of a person's mind or making them do something against their will. By this definition hypnosis doesn't work, yet as you've learned, that isn't how hypnosis really works at all.

The second thing that makes this myth prevalent is the previously discussed lack of training by many practicing hypnotherapists. Because they are trained in a limited number of styles and skills, while at the same time promoting unrealistic one-session cures for complex conditions, this frequently leads to them over-promising and under-delivering. This in turn leaves many people who've had experience with these hypnotists with the opinion that hypnosis doesn't work. But what is the reality of the efficacy of hypnosis?

The reality is hypnosis is an incredibly powerful healing modality that has been used for thousands of years and is endorsed by major medical associations around the world. It's a commonly unknown fact that many surgeries around the world are done completely pain-free using only hypnosis in instances where the patient is allergic to anesthesia or simply wants a natural approach. Try telling one of these people who had surgeons cut into them with no anesthesia, yet felt no pain, that hypnosis doesn't work. Let's look at some statistics.

One of the larger and more frequently cited studies was one in which 2,000 cumulative studies and articles on hypnosis/hypnotherapy, cognitive behavioral therapy, and on psychoanalysis were compared. The study was focused on determining long-term success rates. The study determined the following:

Behavioral Therapy had a 72% success rate after 22 sessions.

Psychotherapy had a success rate of 38% after an average of 600 sessions.

Hypnotherapy had a 93% success rate after only 6 sessions.

These statistics speak for themselves. My personal belief is that if the study excluded all case studies by hypnotherapists with less than 1000 hours of training as well as hypnotherapists with less flexibility because of being trained in only one modality or style (classical, Ericksonian, etc.) the success rate of hypnosis would have been substantially higher than 93%.

Hypnotherapy and hypnosis has been instrumental to the amazing weight loss results I have helped clients achieve, and the principles underlying Clinical Hypnotherapy are a major part of the foundation of the *Fat to Fearless*® program.

You may know people who have tried hypnosis for weight loss, but they did not achieve success. It is important to understand that the type of hypnotherapy used as well as the level of the practitioner's training and credentials play a large role.

Most hypnotherapists who practice with the minimum required level of education are only trained in what is called suggestion therapy. During suggestion therapy, the client is put into a light to medium level of hypnosis and given instructions of how they will be different. Instructions such as "you are now fully satisfied after your last meal of the evening" or "you now enjoy eating healthy food" are said to the client while they are in the trance state. At best, this type of hypnotherapy works only in the short term. This is because it does little to resolve the underlying core beliefs and only focuses on the symptoms of overeating. You've already learned why exclusively focusing on the symptoms doesn't work in the long run. Interactive Clinical Hypnotherapy is the most effective way to use hypnosis to produce permanent results.

During Interactive Clinical Hypnotherapy, the client is not just spoken too by the therapist, but speaks back and actively participates. This allows the therapist to dialogue directly with the client's subconscious mind to create amazing transformations in each session.

If you have the full *Fat to Fearless*® program, you received a series of Hypnotherapy Audio Sessions with complete instructions on how to use them. If you only purchased the book and would like to get the full program, please visit:

www.fattofearless.com

This book, along with the *Fat to Fearless*® Hypnotherapy Audio Sessions and the Success Guide and Workbook, combine the best parts of suggestion therapy, cognitive restructuring, and Interactive Clinical Hypnotherapy to produce amazing results without live sessions. Unlike in live sessions, the workbook and exercises will allow your own conscious mind to take the place of the therapist to process what is uncovered in your audio hypnosis sessions. This is why following through on all of the components of the program is so important. They are more than the sum of their parts and work together to transform the subconscious issues that have been holding you back. While live sessions in my office or through Skype are the fastest way to produce results, the interactive media program when combined with the workbook will get you to your goal as well.

Information on in-person sessions and group coaching can be obtained at:

www.asherfoxweightloss.com/personalsessions
www.asherfoxweightloss.com/groupcoaching

EXERCISE: HYPNOTHERAPY AUDIO SESSIONS

When you purchase the full *Fat to Fearless*® program you received a series of Hypnotherapy Audio Sessions. These sessions were designed for you to begin using at the beginning of the program. If you haven't already done so, please read the instructions that accompany them and begin using them daily.

SUMMARY

Key Points

- Hypnosis is defined as a natural, yet altered state of mind where the Critical Gateway is bypassed and there is access to the subconscious mind.

- The "trance state" is a natural state you go in and out of several times a day. Becoming absorbed in an activity or television show where you lose awareness of your surroundings is one example. Another example is arriving somewhere and not remembering all the details of the drive. In this instance, your subconscious mind took over and did the driving for you while your conscious mind was otherwise engaged.

- One definition of hypnosis, given by famed hypnotherapist and medical doctor Milton Erickson, is that "hypnosis is a state of learning." This definition makes even more sense when we understand that any learning that stays with us must involve the subconscious mind.

- Accessing the hypnotic state and gaining access to the unconscious mind makes available to you the nearly unlimited resources of the subconscious to create lasting change in your life.

- One of the biggest challenges with hypnosis in modern society is the many myths and misperceptions people have about it. Reviewing those myths in this chapter and understanding the truth about hypnosis will allow you to consciously understand how useful and effective hypnosis will be on your *Fat to Fearless®* journey.

- No one can be made to do something in hypnosis that violates their moral principles.

- Hypnosis is not like being asleep. The dual nature of the mind is such that any time you are actually awake both your conscious and subconscious minds are present to some degree.

- Since you are actually following the hypnotherapist's instructions in your own mind, you are effectively hypnotizing yourself. All hypnosis is "self-hypnosis," and anyone can be hypnotized if they're willing to commit themselves to the process and find a well-trained and experienced hypnotherapist.

- Only in rare instances is hypnosis a single session cure. For most lifelong issues, like chronic weight problems, multiple sessions are required. This is why the *Fat to Fearless*® program includes multiple audio sessions designed to be used over time as you move through different sections of the program.

- Being able to be hypnotized has nothing to do with having a weak mind. In fact, the best hypnotic subjects are ones who can easily follow instructions and have creative minds.

- Studies have shown that hypnosis, when used by qualified and experienced hypnotherapists, has a significantly higher success rate over other types of therapies.

- Hypnotherapy works in conjunction with everything you've learned about the subconscious mind, including the power of repetition, to create lasting change. For the *Fat to Fearless*® Hypnotherapy Audio Sessions to be effective you must consistently use them over the amount of time suggested in the instructions they came with.

- The fastest way to create the subconscious changes that allow you to lose weight and keep it off is with private sessions in my Orlando office or by enrolling in one of my online group coaching programs. However, by going through the program yourself you can still produce the necessary changes at a slower pace.

- Information on in-person sessions and group coaching can be obtained at:

  www.asherfoxweightloss.com/personalsessions
  www.asherfoxweightloss.com/groupcoaching

What This Has To Do With Weight Loss

Creating lifelong change in your body, your eating habits, and the emotions that are intertwined with them requires creating change at the subconscious level. Hypnotherapy, when used by an experienced and well-trained professional, is one of the fastest and most effective ways to do exactly that.

Hypnosis and its underlying principles drive much of the neural change technology embedded in the *Fat to Fearless*® Hypnotherapy Audio Sessions.

You Are Ready To Move To The Next Chapter When . . .

- You have an understanding of the reality of what hypnosis is versus the myths and misconceptions perpetuated by television and fiction.

- You have watched the tutorial video for this chapter (if you have the full *Fat to Fearless*® program).

- You have begun using the Hypnotherapy Audio Sessions as per their included instructions (if you have the full *Fat to Fearless*® program).

CHAPTER 13

BYPASSING THE CRITICAL GATEWAY WITH VISUALIZATION AND EMOTION

Opening The Critical Gateway: Changing Your Subconscious Body Image

As you learned in the last chapter, hypnosis is one way to bypass the Critical Gateway. Another is visualization. Visualization, for our purposes, is defined as creating an internal representation of an experience that you'd like to have.

The subconscious mind, to the degree imagined events are "emotionalized," can't distinguish it from real events. The term emotionalized means "imagined in a way that produces an emotional response." Therefore, using a combination of emotion, visualization, and repetition you can begin reprogramming your subconscious mind. Let's see how this pertains to what's called your subconscious body image.

Your subconscious body image is how you see and perceive your body at a deep, subconscious level. Do you see yourself as a fat person? As long as you do, your subconscious will act on that belief to prove you right. This is because "seeing yourself as a fat person" is essentially believing at a subconscious level that you are a fat person. As you remember, the subconscious acts to prove our beliefs true. In this instance, your subconscious acts on your image-belief to sabotage your ability to lose weight and keep it off.

To be successful with long-term weight loss you must change your subconscious body image to match the body you consciously want. When you change your subconscious body image to that of the body you desire you are aligning your conscious and subconscious minds to get results. Your secret weapon in changing your subconscious body image will be your imagination.

Neville Goddard, the 20th-century leader of the New Thought movement, was one of the first modern proponents of the mind's ability to create its own reality through the use of your imagination when he coined the term "imaginal" living. Since then, countless others have elaborated on this belief, and in varying degrees the study of quantum physics has also supported your mind's ability to create new circumstances in your outer world by first pre-designing them in your inner world.

In the past decade there has been a lot of attention around the Law of Attraction, which is the idea that "like attracts like." By imagining your circumstances as you want them to be in an emotional way, you become "like" what you are trying to attain and thus draw it to you. There are as many skeptics as proponents of these theories, yet for many they do seem to work. The reason that many refuse to believe in the Law of Attraction, in spite of plenty of anecdotal evidence that it works, is that it seems too much like "magic" or pseudo-science.

It's true that much of the material available today related to the Law of Attraction is based on a biased and at most cursory understanding of the principles underlying true quantum physics. It's also true, however, that most who consistently apply its principles produce results. Let's clear up the mystery around the Law of Attraction so that you can use this tool to help you achieve permanent weight loss without feeling as if you are relying on magic. The reason The Law of Attraction (emotionally visualizing what you want to draw into your life) is successful and works has more to do with how the process affects the subconscious mind as it does anything else.

The reason that consistently imagining what you want in an emotional way is so powerful is because of the principles of the subconscious mind that you've already learned. Regardless of metaphysics, these internal imaginings create your reality by reprogramming the subconscious mind and the Reticular Activating System (R.A.S.) to bring your imagined reality to pass.

You've already learned that any new activity or habit requires the brain to build new neural pathways to enable these new experiences. Fortunately, these experiences can be imagined before they actually happen. Remember, the subconscious mind does not know the difference between events that are emotionally imagined and real happenings. This allows you to use visualization to build the neurological structures in your mind that support long-term weight loss.

For example, let's say that you have a hard time going to the gym after work. By using the principles taught in this chapter you could create an imagined scene, infused with motivating emotion, in which you excitedly go to the gym after work and enjoy the positive results you get from working out. As you continue to imagine those events in detail and with emotion, your brain will respond by building the neural pathways that correspond to that activity. The result: with the neural pathways already built, and the positive motivating emotions already built into them, you will find it easier to actually follow through with your after-work exercise in the real world.

A great metaphor for understanding this process is being in the jungle and wanting to travel to a new destination. To get where you want to go you're going to need to cut a path through the jungle. This certainly decreases your motivation to undertake the journey. Hacking through the jungle, creating a new path to a new destination, is like building new neural pathways to new activities.

You would be much more likely to undertake your jungle trip if the path was already built. However, if you could simply imagine yourself cutting a path through the foliage and the jungle responded by creating that path on its own, that would make it easier as well. Under these circumstances you would have far less mental resistance to beginning your jungle trek.

In this metaphor, the jungle is your brain, the path is your neural pathways, and the new destination is your weight loss goal. By imagining yourself engaging in the activities that support you in losing weight and keeping it off, you're creating the mental pathways to make it easier to follow through in the physical world.

Effective use of your imagination can help you drop the pounds in the "real" world as easily as you can in your mental reality. The first use of your imagination to help you reach these goals is to build a new subconscious body image through imagined experience.

Even though his technique is often referred to as visualization, it isn't always pictures that you "see." For many, their sense of smell, touch, or just emotional impressions take center stage in their "imaginings." Regardless of your natural inclination, the more senses you can involve, the closer these imagined experiences will come to replicating real life. Subsequently, the more your imaginings mirror reality, the more your brain is convinced that these imagined experiences are real and responds by building new associations and neural pathways.

The first step in this process is to create a mental image of how you want your body to look when you reach your goal weight. It's important that this image be believable and realistic for you, otherwise it could bring up feelings of doubt. If you find this is the case for you, then visualizing an intermediate goal that you will later update as you make progress may be best.

Next, you will create a specific scene where you have already reached your goal weight and are experiencing having the body you want. You can use your positive life story that you wrote at the beginning of the book for inspiration; however, this scene you create will be more focused and have more detail. Think of it as a five-minute trailer for the movie of your life after weight loss. Let's Get Stared.

EXERCISE: NEW BODY "MOVIE TRAILER"

In this exercise you are going to create a "movie trailer" of you living life with the new body you're on your way to achieving. Movie trailers are the previews you see of upcoming films at the theater. Movie trailers show the very best parts of a movie in an attempt to make the viewers feel emotions that motivate them to see the film. You are going to do the same thing.

In this exercise, your New Body Movie Trailer is going to be designed to create the emotions in you that create motivation while also programming your subconscious to live the experience of having the body featured on your internal movie screen.

Step 1: Create the New You

Create the "you" that is going to be in your New Body Movie Trailer. See your body in detail and exactly as you want it to be. When doing this, it is important to balance realistic expectations with what motivates you. Realistic expectations does not mean limiting the amount of weight you are going to lose but takes into consideration things like age and body type. For instance, at the time I am writing this book I am in my late 30s and have broad shoulders. No matter how much weight I lose, I am never going to have the body of a thin 18-year-old swimmer without changing my bone structure. Also, if you are 78 years old, imagining the body of a 20-year-old may not be realistic either. Envisioning the best possible body for you will create the best results.

Your new imagined body should not be how you are now, but it should also be believable as a body you can achieve. Otherwise, if it's too unbelievable you will activate the Inner Critic, which will continuously tell you that you are never going to get there. This would of course be counter productive to maintaining the best emotional state to get results.

If you have so much weight to lose that your final goal weight is impossible for you to conceive achieving at this time, then imagine your body 30 or 40 pounds less, and update your New Body Movie Trailer as your body continues to change.

Step 2: Mentally Film Your Movie Trailer

Now "film" the five-minute movie trailer of the life you will live after you've reached your goal weight. Just like a Hollywood movie trailer is designed to sell a movie to the audience, this trailer will "sell" the image of your new body to your subconscious. Think about what you now know about your subconscious mind and what it takes for it to "buy in" to things.

You know that your subconscious mind is your emotional mind, so your movie trailer must be filled with highly emotional scenes related to what you will feel when you reach your goals. Also, the subconscious mind only exists in the now, so your movie trailer must be staged as if you have already reached your goals.

Your subconscious mind is also very literal. If you imagine that this is something that is going to happen in the future, that's what will be impressed upon the subconscious mind. Subsequently, you will never reach your goal as your subconscious will follow your instructions by making sure it's always something that is going to happen *in the future*.

Your movie trailer might include scenes like the following:

Seeing yourself looking and feeling amazing while trying on new clothes. As you leave the store, you see you are noticed and looked at as desirable. Before you get out of the store, you are stopped and asked on a date by exactly the type of person you have always believed would be attracted to you if you looked and felt the way you wanted to.

Or...

Maybe it is a scene where you are enjoying time with your family and you notice how your spouse is looking at you in a way that hasn't happened in years. You also enjoy how much energy you have playing with your children. You talk about the exciting vacations you will take where you do more active things now that you are much healthier, and have much more stamina and energy.

Perhaps it's a scene at work, when a colleague compliments you about how good you look. This occurs just before you step into the front of a meeting room where you give a dynamic presentation with confidence and charisma. You notice how much more in control of yourself you are and how much more respect you get from your peers since you learned to love and respect yourself by taking care of your health and your body.

Your individual scene may not be anything like the ones above, but it must be completely yours and as personal and powerful as you can make it. Also, you want to make sure this scene displays all of your new positive core beliefs in the way that the "story of your life" you wrote in the beginning pointed to the negative ones. You should be able to easily see your new core beliefs in your imagined movie, almost as if they were the moral of the story.

Write your New Body Movie Trailer scene out now either in your *Fat to Fearless®* Success Guide and Workbook or on your own sheet of paper.

Step 3: Add Emotional Editing

You will now take the "raw footage" you just created in your mind and add emotional editing. The reason many people visualize (or imaginalize) and it does not work is because it is not emotional enough. Remember, the two most powerful elements that impact the subconscious mind are repetition and emotion. The more emotional it is, the less repetition it takes. Many people visualize for weeks, months, and years but never really create enough emotion for it to have an impact. Follow the steps below to ensure your New Body Movie Trailer has the most emotional impact possible to reach your subconscious.

1. Review your scene and make sure you have included everything you can to get you excited about reaching your

goal. Are there any symbols that you can include that trigger thoughts of weight loss success?

2. It is a good idea to include not only the end result of the body you want, but also some of the behaviors that created the result. Maybe in the scene where you are trying on those clothes over your great new body you get a text message from a friend confirming your reservations at a healthy eating restaurant, and you take the time to be thankful that you now eat healthy. Include as many positive habits and processes that you can in your scene so that you are also programming in these behaviors while also changing your subconscious body image to match the body you want.

3. Neuro-Linguistic Programming, which is the study of the structure of subjective experience, tells us that when we adjust the details of how we represent things to ourselves in our mind it subsequently affects our emotional states. We will be learning about this in more detail later, but for now we will focus on the visual elements of your movie trailer by having you adjust the visual details to give you maximum emotional effect. To illustrate this concept find a memory of something unpleasant, something that bothers you significantly.

Once you have the image of that memory in your mind, close your eyes and shrink the picture of that memory in your head. Imagine that you are moving it further away. If the picture is in color, turn it to black-and-white and maybe make it grainy and fuzzy. Notice how that affects the way you feel about your memory.

Most people find that the memory loses much of its power when the visual details are adjusted this way. If that didn't work for you, play with all of the visual details until you begin to notice a change in the way the memory makes you feel. On the next page is a list of some of the common visual elements you can adjust.

- Distance or how far away it seems
- Brightness
- Color or black-and-white
- Image size
- Is there a frame or border around the image?
- Sharpness/Fuzziness
- Is the memory a movie or a still frame?
- Location: Where do you "see" the memory in your mind's eye? Is it to the left or right of you? Is it below or above eye level? etc.

Play with all of these elements until you notice you can change the way the unpleasant memory or image makes you feel to have less of a negative impact on you.

The purpose of the above exercise was to demonstrate how changing those elements in the way you internally represent a memory can also change how that memory makes you feel. Just like you can lessen the negative impact of events by changing the visual details, you can also increase your positive feelings about pleasant memories by doing the same in the opposite way.

To illustrate how to increase your positive feelings, choose a moderately pleasant memory and make the memory brighter, closer, or adjust one of the other visual details listed above and notice how it makes you feel.

One important visual detail that I have not included in the list is whether or not you are experiencing the memory as associated or disassociated. Associated means you are seeing this scene as if it is through your own eyes. You are in the memory and it is happening right now. If it is disassociated, you are seeing it as if you are watching yourself, as if on a movie and outside of yourself.

For most people, the memory will have more emotional impact if you are associated with it (seeing it through your eyes as if you are there). However, this does not hold true for everyone. When I created my own New Body Movie Trailer, I found it had more impact when I saw it disassociated so that I could admire my body in the image.

If you find you produce more positive emotion by playing your New Body Movie Trailer as if seeing it through your own eyes, you will need to put some element in the movie, like a mirror or looking at current photos of yourself so you can see the new you while in the scene and begin subconsciously owning your new body.

Also you can create two versions of the movie, one where you are associated and seeing it through your own eyes, and one where you are disassociated as if watching it on a movie screen. Play them both daily. In the movie that is associated, focus on the physical feelings in your body, both your positive emotions as well as things like increased energy and more confident movements. In the disassociated movie, emphasize appreciating the appearance of your body. You will find what works best for you in time.

Now, the last step in the editing process is to go through your scene and adjust the lighting, color, and size of the images. Try it associated and disassociated. Play with all of the other visual elements until you have your New Body Movie Trailer where it creates the strongest positive emotional feelings within you, just like a movie trailer that pushes all the right buttons and pulls all the right heartstrings.

Step 4: Add Multiple Senses

As we've discussed, the subconscious mind perceives emotionally imagined events as real events, and the more real you make it, the more impact it has. Almost every experience in the real world involves multiple senses, so too should your imagined ones.

Go back through your scene and add sounds, smells, and kinesthetic sensations (touch and physical feelings within your body) to your trailer. Perhaps there is a song playing on the radio in your scene that's particularly motivating to you, or maybe there's the smell of saltwater as you step out onto the beach in your new bathing suit that reminds you of how long you've wanted to walk down the beach looking this good.

Physical sensations are also important. Notice how those new clothes feel on your skin. Take time to appreciate how much physically lighter you feel. Notice the way your body feels moving with increased energy and better health.

Smell is often the hardest sense to include. If nothing in your scene lends itself to including a smell, or if the smell would serve no purpose to help make this seem more real for you, it is not necessary to include it.

Definitely try to include both audio and kinesthetic senses in addition to visual. One thing I suggest is to include the sound of a healthier internal voice praising you in the scene. This voice reminds you how great you are and how wonderful it is that you followed through on reaching your goal weight. It praises you for doing it in a way that you can keep it off and live a happy life. In the next section you are going to learn how to create weight loss affirmations personalized for you. These affirmations would be great things for your healthy internal voice to say to you in your scene.

Step 5. Pre-screen Your Trailer

The first step to pre-screen your trailer is to get yourself in a movie-watching mood by getting yourself into a relaxed place with no distractions.

One of the best ways to do this is to listen to the Hypnosis Trance Training Audio Session included in the full *Fat to Fearless*® program. This audio session is designed to put you into a brainwave state that allows you more access to the subconscious mind while also relaxing you. It is also encoded with subliminal weight loss suggestions. If you do not have access to your *Fat to Fearless*® audios, then simply sit and focus on breathing in a slow rhythmic pattern until you feel relaxed.

Once you are relaxed, run your movie with all of the emotional high points, sights, sounds, smells, and physical sensations. Notice how it makes you feel. If you feel excited, energized, and look forward to the future when you reach your weight loss goal because it feels like it is right there in front of you right now, then your trailer is a success! It is ready to sell your subconscious on the new movie of your life starring your new body image where you look great, feel amazing, and are living life to its fullest. If you did not get that effect, re-run these steps until you create, edit, and adjust your trailer to produce that strong positive emotional effect. You'll know when it's perfect for you.

Step 6: Play Your Trailer Multiple Times Every Day

Now that you have your emotionalized New Body Movie Trailer ready, you want to show it to your audience (your subconscious) as often as possible so it will buy into the movie (your new subconscious body image) and adopt these images and the beliefs around them as true. You do this in three ways:

1. Before falling asleep each night, play the scene in your mind at least once with as much positive emotion as possible. Do the same thing again every morning upon waking. If you are using your *Fat to Fearless*® Hypnotherapy Audio Sessions at night, each session gives you time to visualize. Your New Body Movie Trailer is the perfect visualization for this time.

2. Whenever you have time during the day, even if you don't have access to the hypnosis audios, play your trailer with emotion.

3. During most all of the *Fat to Fearless*® Hypnotherapy Audio Sessions there will come a time when I will ask you to play out your ideal scene or imagine having already reached your goals. These are excellent times in the session to plug this scene in.

Do this exercise throughout the *Fat to Fearless*® process until you reach your goal weight. Then update your movie with new goals! New research has shown that it takes 66 days to form a habit (asherfoxweightloss.com/habits). Commit to playing your trailer for at least 66 days and within 30 days you will already notice powerful changes happening. You will be amazed at the difference in your self-esteem and self-perception on Day 66.

*If you have trouble with this exercise because you have strong negative emotions about your body, or specific parts of your body, clearing these negative emotions before this exercise is very helpful. Please visit the following webpage for additional information on how to eliminate any strong negative feelings you have about your appearance before doing this exercise:

www.asherfoxweightloss.com/bodyimage

SUMMARY

Key Points

- To the degree an imagined experience is "emotionalized" (produces an emotional response), the subconscious mind can't differentiate between it and a real event.

- Using the above principle, you can use visualization, emotion, and repetition to reprogram the subconscious mind.

- Your subconscious body image is how you see and perceive your body at a deep and subconscious level.

- If your subconscious body image is that of a fat person, your subconscious perceives this as a core belief. It will act on that image to prove you right and ensure you stay overweight by ensuring your body matches that image in your mind.

- To achieve long-term weight loss, you must change your internal subconscious body image to match the body you want so your subconscious works to help you attain that body.

- Your best weapon in changing your subconscious body image is your imagination.

- Repeatedly imagined experiences create corresponding neural pathways that make the activity easier in real life. For example, imagining yourself enjoying going to the gym will create neural structures that make it easier to follow through in the real world.

- Even though this technique is often called "visualization," it isn't always pictures that you see. For many, these imagined experiences are felt most strongly through their other senses.

- The more of your senses (sight, sound, taste, touch, smell) you involve in your imagined experiences, the more your subconscious perceives them as real.

- A New Body Movie Trailer is a great way to begin transforming your subconscious body image to one that supports you in reaching your weight loss goals.

What This Has To Do With Weight Loss

Your subconscious constructs your body, in part, based on your internalized unconscious image of yourself. Changing this subconscious body image to match your weight loss goals is paramount to enlisting the aid of your subconscious in reaching those goals in the physical world.

You Are Ready To Move On When . . .

- You understand you have an internal unconscious body image that your subconscious acts on like a core belief. Like all core beliefs, your subconscious wants to prove this image to be true and therefore works to ensure your outer body corresponds to this internal image.

- You understand how visualization, emotion, and repetition work together to allow you to program in a new subconscious body image that works with you toward helping you reach your weight loss goals.

- You have watched the tutorial video for this chapter (if you have the full *Fat to Fearless*® program).

- You have completed the exercises for this chapter in the Success Guide and Workbook (if you have the full *Fat to Fearless*® program).

CHAPTER 14

BYPASSING THE CRITICAL GATEWAY
WITH EMOTIONALIZED AFFIRMATIONS

Opening The Critical Gateway:
Emotionalized Affirmations

In the last two chapters, you learned about hypnosis and visualization as ways to bypass the Critical Gateway. The third way is with emotionalized affirmations. We are impacted by the words that are said about us. Whether it be about our bodies, our intellects, our past, our cultural heritage or anything else related to our "self-hood." However, we are especially impacted by those words that are already consistent with our existing core beliefs. Because these words resonate with our secret fears about ourselves, they go straight through the Critical Gateway and into the subconscious. But as powerful as what others say to us can be, it is the things we say to ourselves that have the most impact.

It is that critical voice in our head, the Inner Critic that you've already learned about, that does so much to keep us stuck in the lives we've created from our limiting core beliefs. When teaching hypnotherapy students I often ask them which is worse, the real-life negative events of childhood or the Inner

Critic that evolves from them. They quickly learn that the answer is the Inner Critic, because long after the real-life abuse stops, the Inner Critic is still going strong with its negative assessments and criticisms. Without intervention, the voice of the Inner Critic lasts a lifetime.

The good news is that you can interrupt the voice of the Inner Critic from force-feeding you negative thoughts by choosing to nourish yourself with positive ones. However, you need to develop these positive thoughts in advance if they are going to be successfully used when you need them the most. In a future chapter we will deal with actually dismantling the voice of the Inner Critic, but for now we are going to create the new healthier voice that will take its place.

The reason you need to develop positive thoughts in advance is because they are not yet habit for you. In the heat of the moment of an event that normally creates self-criticism, without those positive thoughts ready for action, the delay will give the Inner Critic the time to interject its negative self-talk and do its job of making you feel bad to keep you in line with your negative beliefs.

Your goal is to stop the negative thoughts of the Inner Critic, replace them with emotionally positive statements, and do this before you are negatively affected by the Inner Critic. Without a plan to implement in advance, it is far too easy to slip back into your old self-condemning habits. For our purposes, we will call these positive thoughts affirmations.

To affirm something means to declare it as true. Some people have an issue with affirmations because they feel they are lying to themselves if they feel these statements are not yet true. I respond to that with a question. Is the seed of an oak tree lying to itself by saying it is a tree, or does it simply recognize its potential? I want you to view affirmations as who you would already be if your negative core beliefs had not gotten in your way.

While this may not change your feeling right away that your affirmations aren't quite true, in time the repetition of practicing your affirmations will take effect, and you will feel as if they are more true every day. Eventually you will feel as if your affirmations are true, and you will notice how your subconscious recreates your life in accordance with your affirmations.

In the meantime, that feeling of dissonance that what you are saying in these affirmations does not match your current reality is a tool that you can actually use to aid you in the process. Let me explain.

As you create and then practice your affirmations, you will use this sense of cognitive dissonance (discomfort from trying to hold two conflicting beliefs) as a guide to see where you have the most work to do. The affirmations that produce the strongest dissonance are where you need to do the most work. As this internal conflict subsides, it is a valuable indicator that you are healing your emotional wounds, the same wounds that lead to being overweight. It is also an indicator that your subconscious is accepting your new beliefs as true.

Another powerful way this sense of cognitive dissonance helps you on your journey is that it makes it harder to engage in unwanted behaviors because it puts a spotlight on them. Previously, when you ate unhealthy you may not have given it a lot of thought until afterwards. It happened in the moment and it was only afterwards that the guilt and shame set in (even though it was there before unconsciously driving the behaviors through the mechanism of the Symptom Cycle).

When you repeat your affirmations throughout the day, you constantly program your conscious and subconscious. An affirmation like "I eat the right foods, in the right amounts, at the right times," puts the thought of the desired behavior in front of you where you can't ignore it. This will either give you the strength to resist, or as you repeatedly give in, the incongruence between declaring these affirmations and your behaviors will cause increasing discomfort. Eventually, this discomfort grows until the pain of giving in to the behavior becomes greater than the perceived pleasure and you stop doing it.

Both consciously and subconsciously, through both the feelings of these affirmations becoming true and the feelings of cognitive dissonance created in the beginning of this process, affirmations are a powerful tool on your journey. But what makes affirmations work for some and not for others?

What makes affirmations powerful tools for some, yet ineffective for others is how well these affirmations are designed. The better they are designed, the better they can go through the Critical Gateway and reach the subconscious mind. Again, repetition and emotion are very important. The more emotionally charged your affirmation is, the less repetition that is needed for it to impact the subconscious mind. For many, affirmations do not work because they do not have enough emotional charge embedded in them and the amount of repetition is too low to make up for it.

The key is to create affirmations that are charged with the positive emotions you know you want to feel once you reach your goal. Then, combine that with as much repetition as possible. How long it takes for affirmations to create change is based on how emotional they are, how often you repeat them, what other techniques and tools you are combining with them, and the level of subconscious resistance. Because you are listening to your *Fat to Fearless*® Hypnotherapy Audio Sessions while also doing the other exercises and work throughout the program, there will be a synergistic effect that increases the power of your affirmations and how fast they work.

The following exercises help you create and use your *Fat to Fearless*® affirmations.

1. Create your affirmations using transformational language.

2. Make sure your affirmations pass the "believability test."

3. Set up your delivery system.

EXERCISE: CREATE YOUR AFFIRMATIONS

It's now time to create your affirmations. Your affirmations will be very personal and powerful statements about you, about your capabilities and behaviors, or about the specific results and outcomes they produce. Let's look at these three types of affirmations.

Affirmations about "you" are what you believe about yourself and can be the verbatim core beliefs you want to adopt to replace your negative core beliefs. Examples may be, *I am more than good enough* or *I am lovable and deserve the best life has to offer.*

Affirmations about outcomes and results are things you do not directly control, but are the results of your behaviors and actions. *I now lose one or more pounds every week* or *I now have more energy every day* would be good examples. You do not directly control these things. There is no button you push to lose weight or lever you pull to adjust how energetic you feel. They are the result of healthy habits.

Affirmations about behaviors are specific actions you will take that support both your new core beliefs and the desired outcomes (losing weight and keeping it off). Examples might be, *I now enjoy exercising three or more days a week* or *I eat the right foods in the right amounts at the right times.*

When you create your affirmations, you will have at least one affirmation at each of the above three levels. For example, if one of your negative core beliefs is that you are unlovable, you might create the positive affirmation that says "I am lovable."

You would also have an affirmation about the behaviors that supports your belief that you are lovable. Acts of self-love might include spending five minutes each day to list your positive qualities or keeping a gratitude journal or any activity related to better physical and mental health, such as eating better, exercising, or meditation.

Last, you will include an affirmation about the results you expect to receive from believing you are lovable and engaging in activities that affirm that to you. One example might be, "I now attract people into my life that love, honor, and respect me." You can't directly control who comes into your life, but this would be an expected outcome of adopting this positive belief and acting in accordance with it.

Here are some guidelines for creating your affirmations using transformational language.

1. **Be positive.** Affirmations should be statements of what you want, not what you do not want. As an example, you would not want to say, *I am not fat.* Instead you would say, *I am thin, healthy, and happy!*

   It's often said that the subconscious doesn't perceive negatives and if you were to have an affirmation that said *I will not overeat,* your subconscious doesn't "hear" the negative word *not* and will only "hear" *I will overeat.* This actually isn't correct as the subconscious certainly hears all of the words, positive and negative. The reason you do not want to use negatives when constructing affirmations has to do with another way in which the subconscious mind interprets input.

   The subconscious operates at a broader level than the conscious mind. It is not as concerned with the details of something as it is with what it is about. The statement, *I am not fat* to the subconscious mind is not about losing weight, but about being fat, so it reinforces in the subconscious the idea of being fat. It's similar to the concept of "don't think of a purple elephant." You cannot think about "not being fat" without also thinking about "being fat." Essentially, being fat is the subject of the affirmation.

   Inversely, affirmations about not being thin, happy, and healthy are still about being thin, happy and healthy.

The bottom line is that the subconscious will respond to the subject of the affirmation, to what it is about. Make the subject of your affirmations what you want to be, do and have instead of what you are trying to avoid.

2. **Be in the now.** All of your affirmations should be stated in the present because the subconscious mind operates in the present moment and does not understand the concepts of past and future. For example, you would not want to say, *I will lose weight*, because it implies it is something you will do in the future. The subconscious mind takes things very literally. If you say you "will" lose weight, your subconscious will always keep it as something that is going to happen in the future, not something that is happening now. Instead say, *I easily lose weight now!*

3. **Do not imply ability.** Again, the subconscious mind is very literal, and implying the ability to do something does not mean you will do it. If you think about it, you know this is true in your conscious mind as well. You know how to lose weight. You have probably done it many times, so you know you have the ability to do it. Despite this ability, however, you have not lost weight and kept it off. For this reason, avoid using words like "can" or "ability." For example, do not say, *I can easily exercise 30 minutes every day* or *I have the ability to easily lose weight.* Instead say, *I now easily exercise 30 minutes every day* or *I now easily lose weight.*

4. **Be specific.** This will not be true for all affirmations, but whenever possible, create your affirmations in a way that is not vague and also matches your goal with a time frame. For example, *I now easily lose two or more pounds every week* is specific and measurable.

5. **Keep it short and simple.** Think of the subconscious mind like a small child that only grasps simple concepts. Avoid

creating your affirmations with complex sentences. Keep them short and simple.

6. **Use many powerful and personal words that trigger your positive emotions.** For example, if words like "sexy," "hot," "fit," or "firm" create an emotionally motivating response for you, be sure to use them.

Now that you know the transformational language of affirmations, it is time to write yours. Be sure that your affirmations are not only compatible with but also reinforce your new core beliefs that you are installing into your subconscious. You can actually use your new desired core beliefs as affirmations, such as *I am more than good enough, I am perfect, whole, and complete*, etc.

Following is a list of pre-made affirmations that you can use as examples or adopt as your own exactly as they are written. Be sure to include some that are specific to weight loss and some that specifically reinforce your new core beliefs.

Create or choose from five to no more than eight affirmations.

If you would like to have me review the affirmations you've created to make sure they are worded to produce the most powerful subconscious results, or would like to have me create custom affirmations for you based on a telephone or Skype session, please visit: www.asherfoxweightloss.com/affirmations

PRE-MADE WEIGHT LOSS AFFIRMATIONS

Weight Loss Affirmations

On or before (goal date) I now weigh (goal weight) or less.

I eat the right foods, in the right amounts, at the right times.

I enjoy exercising three or more times every week.

I easily release, let go, and lose two or more pounds every week (insert your specific goal).

Every day I am becoming more aware of the relationship between my emotions, food, and my desire to eat.

Awareness is setting me free to have the body I choose to now have.

I now enjoy exercising. The more I exercise the better I feel, and the better I feel the more I exercise.

My metabolism now automatically increases every day. I burn more calories every day—even at night while I sleep.

I now easily stay satisfied after my last meal until breakfast the next morning.

Affirmations About Self

Every day I love myself more as I realize that I am more than good enough and deserve the best life has to offer.

I become more calm, comfortable, and at peace with myself every day.

I love myself and only attract positive people into my life who love me as well.

Every day I learn to love myself more as I acknowledge my beauty both inside and out.

I now take time every day to appreciate and love myself by acknowledging my many positive qualities.

EXERCISE: BELIEVABILITY CHECK

At this point, you should have a list of affirmations you've made for yourself. Now we want to check them to make sure they are not so unbelievable that your Inner Critic so strongly disagrees with them that it fights back and makes it harder for your affirmations to bypass the Critical Gateway and reach your subconscious.

As you've learned one of the ways of getting through the Critical Gateway and reaching the subconscious mind is through repetition. You're going to be using these affirmations in conjunction with your *Fat to Fearless*® Hypnotherapy Audio

Sessions which will use the hypnotic state to bypass the Critical Gateway. However, you will also be using them outside of hypnosis and we want to make sure they are designed in the best possible way to create the least resistance from the Inner Critic and require the least amount of repetition before they begin to take effect.

Step 1

Say each of your affirmations out loud and determine how much internal resistance you have in response. Internal resistance usually comes in the form of the Inner Critic telling you that "it's impossible," "you don't deserve it," "you won't succeed," etc.

For example, if you weigh 300 pounds and your goal weight is to be 160 pounds, telling yourself "I now weigh 160 pounds" might seem so unbelievable that your Inner Critic immediately responds with "Yeah Right!" Instead of it producing a positive feeling, the affirmation instead makes you feel worse and feeds into the Symptom Cycle we discussed, making you possibly want to soothe those bad feelings with food.

We've discussed how these negative feelings about your affirmation not being true can be used to your advantage to let you know where you need to focus on improving the most, but only to an extent. While it's okay if these affirmations don't necessarily feel true now, you do at least need to believe that they are possible. Otherwise, even with repetition they will either never reach your subconscious mind or will take far longer than is practical to get through the Critical Gateway.

Step 2

For each affirmation that feels completely unbelievable and subsequently produces a negative response, try one of the following approaches:

If it's a specific goal, such as weight, choose an intermediate goal that's more believable. Using the above example, instead of programming into your subconscious your final goal weight, you may choose to program in a 20-pound weight loss. While even a 20-pound weight loss may not feel "true" now, it is believable that you can reach it, and with repetition your subconscious mind will accept it as true. Once you've reached the first goal, you will be empowered to set the next one.

Make it incremental. Sometimes, saying that you are a particular way that you know you aren't feels so untrue that it produces such a negative response from the Inner Critic that it is counterproductive. For example, if you are at a point in your life where you are extremely down on yourself and full of self-loathing, an affirmation that states, "I now completely love myself in every way," would feel completely untrue and have little chance of bypassing the Critical Gateway and reaching the subconscious, even with an incredible amount of repetition. The key to this is to make it incremental.

As opposed to stating that you already are whatever it is you are wanting to become, rewrite the affirmation to indicate that you are becoming more that way every day. Using the above affirmation as an example, you might reword it to say "Every day I am learning to love myself more as I acknowledge my many positive qualities." When rephrased this way it produces less of a negative push–back from the Inner Critic and with repetition it will more easily bypass the Critical Gateway.

Step 3

Use the believability test for all of your affirmations and rewrite them as necessary using the above guidelines. When you are done, transfer these affirmations into the appropriate workbook page in your *Fat to Fearless*® Success Guide and Workbook.

EXERCISE: SETUP YOUR SUBCONSCIOUS DELIVERY SYSTEM

Affirmations are used both in and out of hypnosis to help reprogram your subconscious mind. The effectiveness of affirmations is based on how well they are linguistically structured, how emotionally charged they are, and how much repetition you are using to expose them to the subconscious mind. Now that you have created your affirmations it's time to set up how to deliver them to your subconscious using repetition. Your delivery system focuses on repetition.

1. Take your affirmations and put them on a series of index cards. You need five sets: one set for home, one set for work, one set for in your car, and one set to keep with you at all times. In just a moment I'll explain what to do with the fifth set of affirmations.

2. Set a timer (most phones have timers) to remind you at regular intervals to use your set of affirmation cards to say the affirmations to yourself. Since you have a set of affirmation cards at home, work, in your car, and on you at all times, there should never be a reason you can't follow through. Generate as much positive emotion as you can while saying the affirmations. Adjust your internal voice to one of confidence and self-assuredness, and imagine reaching your goals while generating as many positive feelings as possible while saying your affirmations to yourself.

3. To understand how you will use the last set of index cards, it is important to understand how repetition bypasses the Critical Gateway. Have you ever walked into a room and noticed how loud the air conditioning is? Maybe it was so loud that it was a distraction even from conversation. Within a short period of time, however, you no longer noticed it. Even though the sound of the air conditioner was still going into your subconscious, it was bypassing your conscious mind.

   This is an example of how constant exposure causes something to pass from the conscious mind to the subconscious. As you learned, the part of the Critical Gateway involved in rejecting information that contradicts your existing negative core beliefs is located in the conscious mind. The sound of the air conditioning bypassed your conscious mind, and therefore your Critical Gateway. Through constant repetitive exposure, your conscious mind determined it was unworthy of ongoing attention and focus. You will use this understanding with the last set of index cards.

Take the last set of index cards and tape the cards in your home and car in places where you will see them multiple times throughout the day. Initially you consciously notice them, which is still good for repetition and reinforcing the suggestions, but eventually you stop consciously noticing them and they bypass the Critical Gateway and go into your subconscious.

Some examples of places to tape these cards are:

- bathroom mirror
- kitchen cabinets
- refrigerator
- doors
- car (by clock)

4. The next step in your delivery system is to input the affirmations into the Asher Fox Subliminal Belief Software System. If you have not downloaded it already, you can get the program at:

www.asherfoxweightloss.com/software

Follow the software's instructions and once downloaded and installed, it will flash your affirmations on your computer screen at a rate too fast for your conscious mind to notice, which is perfect for your subconscious mind to pick up. Every time you are in front of your computer you will be programming your new positive affirmations and healthier beliefs into your subconscious.

5. The last step in your affirmation delivery system also involves your computer. I discovered by accident how powerful this step is. When I initially created this technique, I did not realize how effective it was until about a month later when I noticed significant improvements in an issue I was working on myself. I knew this one technique was responsible because it was the only thing in my life that had changed.

Take the one affirmation that you consider to be the most important and shorten it so that you can use it for all of your online passwords. Then change every password that you have to this affirmation. While it may be longer or less convenient than your existing passwords, after a week you will no longer notice. Once I did this, I realized that anywhere from 20 to 30 times a day, every time I logged into anything, I was programming this affirmation into my subconscious mind. After about a month I was amazed at the difference it made. Below are a few pointers on how to do this:

If a password requires a number, try using 1 instead of "I" or 0 instead of "o".

If the password requires a symbol, try adding a "!" for emphasis or using a "!" in place of a 1.

Some examples include:

- 1LoveMe

- 1LoseWeightNow!

- 1AmL0vable!

At first, you will be consciously aware that you are typing in this affirmation, but as time goes by you won't even be thinking about what you're typing or its content. At this point, just like the sound of the air conditioner mentioned above, you will be programming into your subconscious your password–affirmation every time you type it.

SUMMARY

Key Points

- Words have more power to impact us than we realize. Specifically, words that confirm our negative core beliefs bypass the Critical Gateway and affect us the most strongly.

- The Inner Critic that develops out of negative experiences in childhood is worse than the actual experiences themselves because the negative voice continues long after the actual events.

- It's important to develop in advance the positive thoughts you use to replace the negative statements of the Inner Critic. This is because the Inner Critic is an automatic response, and if you don't have positive thoughts ready, the negative thoughts will have already been able to do their job of making you feel bad before you can counteract them.

- The positive statements developed for you to use are called affirmations.

- Sometimes affirmations feel difficult because they don't yet feel true. This feeling can be used to highlight where we need to do the most work as well as serve as a gauge to how well our affirmations are working as the feeling of them not being true subsides.

- Affirmations work based on repetition and emotion. The more emotionally charged your affirmations are, the less repetition is necessary for them to affect change in the subconscious mind.

- Your list of affirmations should have statements that affirm your new core beliefs, the behaviors that support those beliefs, and their positive outcome.

- Affirmations must be positive statements phrased in the "now," and don't imply the *ability* to do things but *actually doing them*. They are short and simple and contain as many words as possible that produce powerful positive emotions for you.

- You can actually use your new desired core beliefs verbatim as affirmations.

- You can use word-for-word any of the sample affirmations that seem right for you.

- If an affirmation feels so untrue and unbelievable that it produces a strong negative feeling, either adjust the goal of the affirmation to an intermediate goal or make the change incremental.

- It's important to use all of the steps in the delivery system on a daily basis to ensure that over time and with enough repetition your affirmations produce positive subconscious change that supports you losing weight and keeping it off for a lifetime.

- When you say affirmations aloud, they become declarations. Declarations use the physicality of your body and voice to help align your physiology with your intent.

What This Has To Do With Weight Loss

Affirmations used with the delivery systems described in this chapter will, over time, produce subconscious changes that support you in losing weight and keeping it off. It's important to understand the role repetition plays in affirmations and that the latest research shows it takes 66 days to form a new habit.

It's important to use all aspects of the delivery system with your affirmations for at least 66 days.

You Are Ready To Move On When . . .

- You have created your affirmations and implemented all of the steps in the delivery system to ensure maximum exposure through emotion and repetition to your subconscious mind.

- You have watched the tutorial video for this chapter (if you have the full *Fat to Fearless*® program).

- You have completed the exercises for this chapter in the Success Guide and Workbook (if you have the full *Fat to Fearless*® program).

CHAPTER 15

DEFEAT THE INNER CRITIC

N ow that you are actively at work bypassing your Critical Gateway and programming your subconscious with your new beliefs, it is time for you to consciously overcome your Inner Critic. You've learned that the Inner Critic works to preserve your negative core beliefs and leads to the negative emotions that result in self-sabotaging behaviors. The Inner Critic seems to have a mind of its own. The negative things it says to you seem to arise spontaneously with little choice on your part.

Transforming the Inner Critic is both a conscious and subconscious process. The work you are already doing subconsciously will work to transform the Inner Critic into a positive and healthier voice from the inside out. However, the Inner Critic must also be addressed at the conscious level.

Below are the steps you will take to eliminate the Inner Critic's influence in your life.

1. Determine what the Inner Critic is saying and how it says it.

2. Reverse cognitive distortions.

3. Use humor and affirmations to put the Inner Critic in its place.

The next step in the process is to determine what your Inner Critic says to you that preserves your negative core beliefs. One of the best ways to do this is to use your list of goals and things that you want to do, and then listen to what the Inner Critic has to say about them.

In your next exercise you will do exactly that, but first it's important to understand how to spot the Inner Critic when you hear it.

Identifying the Inner Critic

To change the Inner Critic, you need to know when you hear it speak. Any time you hear the word "should" it is almost always the Inner Critic speaking. "Should" implies a judgment based on an internal set of rules you developed in childhood along with your negative core beliefs. For most of us, this internal set of rules would have us be thin, smart, funny, in control, and financially well off ALL THE TIME. The Inner Critic's list creates a lofty and unrealistic expectation for you. When you do not meet these expectations, the Inner Critic jumps in with the judgments and the "shoulds."

> *You should be thinner.*
>
> *You should take better care of yourself.*
>
> *You should be further along in your life by now.*
>
> *You should be smarter.*
>
> *You should know better.*
>
> *You should be better able to control your eating.*
>
> *You should just* give up.

The list of "shoulds" never stops. On the surface, you can see that this might seem positive. After all, who wouldn't want to be thinner and smarter, etc.? However, the problem lies in the effect these statements produce because they are not about wanting something and going after it, but instead are judgments about how you are deficient for not already having met these goals.

These judgments do not introduce motivating feelings that inspire you to improve your life. Instead, they often make you feel sad, depressed, angry, and all of the other emotions that eventually come out in self-destructive behaviors ranging from binge eating to just giving up. The harsh words of the Inner Critic fuel the Symptom Cycle (the way you feel about being overweight is the indirect cause of the behaviors that keep you overweight).

Another easy way to spot the Inner Critic is any time you find you are putting yourself down or talking to yourself in a way that makes you feel bad. There is a difference between acknowledging you have goals you have not yet reached and berating yourself over not being there yet. One can inspire and move you forward, the other keeps you stuck in the same negative energy that created the very circumstances the Inner Critic is criticizing you for.

In the next exercise you are going to learn to identify the Inner Critic from your other thoughts. If you have the *Fat to Fearless*® Success Guide and Workbook, turn to the appropriate section and do that exercise now. Also, be sure to watch the instructional video related to this exercise. For those of you who only have the book, you can do this exercise on blank sheets of paper.

EXERCISE: INNER CRITIC JOURNAL

Step 1

In the previous exercise "Your Inner Critic Speaks!" you kept a journal where you began identifying the voice of the Inner Critic in your daily life. Now that you have learned more about this voice and have progressed further into the program, you are going to keep this journal for another week so that you have the most up to date information for us to use to begin disempowering the Inner Critic and loosening its hold on you while applying some additional tools as well.

The Inner Critic helps preserve our negative subconscious beliefs. It convinces us that we belong inside the prison of self-sabotage, limited expectations, and negative emotions that those beliefs create for us. It takes both our conscious and subconscious minds to defeat and transform our Inner Critic. We will now focus on becoming consciously aware of what the Inner Critic says to us that impacts us in a way that holds us back.

For the next week, keep a small notebook or your *Fat to Fearless*® Success Guide and Workbook with you throughout the day and write every thought you can attribute to the Inner Critic. You will know these thoughts because they are accompanied by negative feelings.

Write what the Inner Critic actually says, instead of writing *about* what it says. For example, you would not write, *The Inner Critic says bad things to me about me not being good enough and that I'm a loser.* Instead, you would write exactly what it says to you, which may sound like, *You're such a loser. There you go screwing up again. You're so fat, you're never going to lose weight!*

Step 2: Identifying Submodalities

Submodalities is a term used in Neuro-Linguistic Programming (NLP) to describe the different qualities associated with how we represent things to ourselves with our five senses, both internally and externally. Your Inner Critic, for example, is an internal audio representation. That is just a fancy way of saying, *A voice you hear in your head.* The submodalities of that voice are things like:

- volume of the voice

- pitch and tone of the voice

- emotional quality of the voice (does it sound angry, sad, or critical)

- does it feel like it's coming from a particular direction (from in front, behind, etc.)

- any other audio/sound quality

Although it is not actually a submodality, pay attention to identifying if the voice sounds like or reminds you of anyone you know and log that into the appropriate section in your Success Guide and Workbook. Also, be sure to watch the video instructions for this exercise.

I highly recommend doing this for a full week before moving on to the next exercise. Knowing in advance what the next step is will contaminate the quality of your Inner Critic Journal that you need to do first to get the most out of the next exercise. You will however continue to listen to your Hypnotherapy Audio Sessions.

EXERCISE: REVERSE COGNITIVE DISTORTIONS

After completing the last exercise and logging the internal chatter related to your Inner Critic, you should have a better idea of what it says to you, how it says it, and its impact on your life. If you're like most people, this may have been a huge wake up call.

To defeat and transform the Inner Critic, you must never forget this: **the Inner Critic lies.** The things that it tells you about yourself are not true. The negative core beliefs you have about yourself are not true. These are all based on the misperceptions of a child, interpreting things with a child's intellect and emotional immaturity. You then carried the voice of that child with you into adulthood. Remember, the Inner Critic was your worst interpretation of what you heard and experienced growing up as it relates to what was expected of you.

But if the things the Inner Critic says to you are lies, why does it sound so believable to us? To understand this you need to know about cognitive distortions, which are the primary tools the Inner Critic uses to make its lies sound true.

Cognitive Distortions

As you have learned, one of the functions of the subconscious mind is to prove that what you believe about yourself, the world, and the nature of life is true by providing you with evidence that supports those beliefs. You have learned about two important tools used to do that: the Critical Gateway and the Reticular Activating System. But your Inner Critic is also a very powerful tool that aids in that process and has a way of lying to you that makes what it says seem true by using what are called cognitive distortions.

Cognitive distortions are ways that your mind convinces you that something is true that actually is not by linguistically distorting your perception. These inaccurate thought patterns distort, generalize, and delete information within your internal self-talk in a way that has you believing they are true and reinforcing your negative thinking and emotions. They have you telling yourself things that sound rational and accurate on the surface, but really only serve to keep you feeling bad.

Cognitive distortions are distorted thoughts you use to trick yourself into believing your negative thoughts about yourself are accurate. To understand the power of cognitive distortions, it is important to understand the power of language.

Words have the power to affect your emotional state, and your emotional state determines what internal resources you have access to. While it goes beyond the scope of this book, there is a whole science and study dedicated to the connection between how language choice affects our neurology and emotions. Cognitive distortions use language to keep you in an unresourceful state by keeping you in the negative emotions that lead to self-sabotaging behaviors, such as emotional eating or abandoning your weight loss efforts.

The good news is that although cognitive distortions are powerful, once you become conscious of them and challenge them with questions that reveal the truth, they quickly lose their power.

Below is a list of some of the most common cognitive distortions, as well as challenge questions and statements that you can use to disempower them.

1. **Filtering.** When you use the cognitive distortion of filtering, you take the negative details of a situation and focus on them while filtering out all positive aspects. For instance, you may pick out a single, unpleasant detail and dwell on it exclusively so your perception of a situation becomes darkened or distorted. This is not the type of filtering done by the R.A.S. at the neurological level that you are not even aware of. This is filtering done at the conscious level (technically what Freudian psychologists would call the pre-conscious level, but for our purposes we'll refer to it as the conscious level).

   Example: You may have lost three pounds this week, had more energy, and done very well with your eating and exercise, yet you still could not fit into the clothes that you had hoped you could wear this week. The cognitive distortion would be to filter out all of those positive experiences that show you are making great progress and will fit into that clothing soon, and instead focus on not being able to fit into the clothes now. This type of filtering usually leads to a poor emotional state that leads to emotional eating, feeling unmotivated, and making poor decisions about your weight loss program.

   Challenge Questions:
   - What are the positives that I am not thinking about or focusing on?

   - How does only thinking about the negative perpetuate the problem?

   - How will focusing on the positive aspects help me progress faster and farther?

2. **Polarized Thinking (Black-or-White Thinking).** In polarized thinking, things are black-or-white, all-or-nothing. There are no gray areas. You have to be perfect or you are a failure. You either strictly stick to your diet or you binge eat. You place events, people, and situations in either/or categories with no middle ground that allows for how complex most people and situations really are.

If you or anyone else falls short of your expectations, you see yourself, them, or the situation as a total failure. This can obviously lead to the very emotions that cause you to overeat or not exercise. Those who frequently use this cognitive distortion are often prone to periods of binge eating followed by very strict dieting.

Example: You make one small mistake and overeat at one meal, and you feel you have completely blown your diet. This creates the emotional state that leads you to binge eat. Look to identify this cognitive distortion anytime you have had a rapid change in your mood, and ask the challenge questions before you act from your new feelings.

Challenge Questions:

- Am I having an extreme emotional reaction, and if so is it keeping me from seeing the truth about this, which is probably somewhere in the middle?

- What does it really mean when I take the emotion out of it?

- Did I really blow it completely, or is this an overly emotional reaction that will become a self-fulfilling prophecy unless I consciously choose to see this in a more balanced way?

- If the truth about this were really more in the middle, what would that truth be?

3. **Over-Generalization.** Over-generalizations are also known in Neuro-linguistic terms as Universal Quantifiers. In this cognitive distortion, you come to a broad conclusion based on a single situation or piece of evidence. Something occurs once, and you assume that it will continue to happen. One instance can seem as if it is part of an inescapable pattern.

Any time you use the words *always, never, every,* etc., there is usually an over-generalization present. These over-generalizations rob you of being able to form new opinions about new situations, instead causing you to see them through the distortion of old feelings and beliefs.

Example: I always hate to exercise, I never do it right, no one thinks I'm attractive, I always gain the weight back immediately, etc. Over-generalizations, like all cognitive distortions, sound true until you take the time to challenge them.

Challenge Questions:

- Is this really *always* true?

- Has there ever been a time this hasn't been true?

- If there is at least one instance—ever—that this wasn't true, then why am I lying to myself by saying this is always (never, etc.) this way?

- If there is an instance that this hasn't always been true why am I telling myself this lie that makes me feel bad?

- What is the truth of the situation that will help support me in feeling better and reaching my goals?

4. **Mind Reading.** Mind reading is one of the most pervasive and potentially damaging cognitive distortions. Mind reading is when you believe that you know what

others are thinking and proceed from that assumption. The reality is, unless you truly are inside someone's head, you have no idea what they are thinking. Since this cognitive distortion is used by the Inner Critic to help reinforce your existing beliefs, you can rest assured the assumptions you make about others' thoughts are skewed by your own beliefs about yourself.

If you believe you are unworthy, unattractive, not good enough, or have any other limiting belief at a subconscious level, you will assume that people are thinking thoughts that confirm that. Again, this just puts you in an emotional state that activates the Symptom Cycle that leads to self-sabotaging behaviors.

Example: You go to the gym and believe that everyone is looking at you and judging you for your weight, that they are secretly laughing at someone so overweight going to the gym. This is most likely not true, yet it confirms what you secretly believe about yourself because *you judge yourself* in that way. Many clients have told me that after having these thoughts, they feel so self-conscious that after they leave the gym they go home and emotionally eat. A good rule is that anytime you believe you know what someone is thinking about you, it's actually your own projection of what you truly believe about yourself.

The best advice I give clients about mind reading is, if you're going to make up stuff in your head anyway, why not make up stuff that empowers you and makes you feel good!

Challenge Questions:

- Is this actually true?

- What real evidence do I have?

- Can I actually read this person's mind, or is there a chance that what they are actually thinking is something else other than what I fear they are thinking?

- Since I can't actually ready their mind and know what they are thinking, if I'm determined to make something up and believe it's what they are thinking, what would be the best thing I could choose to believe that would best help me in this moment?

5. **Complex Equivalences.** Complex equivalences are when one thing equals another, but you have deleted in your conscious mind the way in which you have made these two things become equal. For example, your significant other may have forgotten to kiss you before leaving for work, so you decided they must be having an affair. You have made one thing equal another, yet you have deleted from your conscious awareness the complex way you used to make these things equivalent.

Usually complex equivalences are combined with other cognitive distortions. For example, *I didn't get the promotion, so my boss must hate me, and I'm sure I'm getting fired.* In this example, mind reading and polarized thinking have been combined to make "not getting the job" equal to "being fired."

Once you question the connection between these two things that often are completely unrelated, it seems ridiculous that you made decisions based on an unconscious correlation designed by your subconscious to keep you engaging in behaviors that reaffirm your existing beliefs.

Example: I looked at that person, and they didn't look back. They must think I'm fat! I've already eaten one chip, I might as well have the whole bag!

Challenge Questions:

- How exactly do those two things equal each other? Why does eating one chip, cookie, etc. mean I should binge eat?

- Is there another reason the person could have not looked back at me other than my weight?

- Are these things always equal or am I making assumptions that support my old limiting beliefs?

6. **Jumping to Conclusions.** Jumping to conclusions is usually combined with mind reading, filtering, polarized thinking, and complex equivalences to allow for reaching a conclusion with limited information. This conclusion usually supports maintaining negative core beliefs. Frequently, this cognitive distortion allows you to reach an incorrect conclusion, after which you do not even bother to get additional information to see if you were correct. You simply treat the conclusion as true and act and feel accordingly.

   Example: My friend Betty started working out and she gained weight, so working out must not be good for women.

   Challenge Questions:

   - Do I have all of the evidence to form a conclusion?

   - How can I better understand what's really going on here?

   - How might this not be true?

7. **Catastrophizing.** In this cognitive distortion, you assume the worst possible outcome no matter how little information you have. You expect problems to strike no matter what. You hear about a problem and use what-if questions (e.g., *What if tragedy strikes? What if it happens to*

me?) to magnify any information that suggests an undesirable outcome, while minimizing signs that things will work out well.

Example: You weigh yourself and even though you lost weight, you did not lose as much as you thought you would. Instead of acknowledging your progress, you jump to the conclusion that your diet is not working and you are not going to reach your goals. This frequently will put you in an emotional state that leads to emotional eating or just wanting to give up, making your "catastrophe" a self-fulfilling prophecy.

Challenge Questions:

- Am I assuming the worst possible thing?

- What evidence do I have that this is true?

- How can I look at this in a more balanced, less emotional way and make a plan for a better outcome?

8. **Personalization.** Personalization is a distortion that relies on another cognitive distortion: mind reading. With personalization, a person believes that everything is about, caused by, or based on them in some way. If someone walks into the office in a bad mood, they must be mad at them. If a friend forgets to call, it must be that they don't care about them.

   Personalization is almost always combined with complex equivalences and mind reading. This cognitive distortion, when combined with the others, allows you to feel personally responsible for everything in your environment that you see as bad or unpleasant. It also supports a victim mentality because it leads you to believe that everything is being done "to you." Using this cognitive distortion is a hallmark of maintaining low self-esteem.

Example: Your friend, who is also on a diet, seems to be avoiding you. You assume it must be because you are setting such a bad example with your own weight loss. This makes you feel worse, which in turn causes you to eventually turn to self-sabotaging behavior.

Challenge Questions:

- What reason do I have to believe that this is about me?

- Am I using mind reading to feel this way?

- What is another possible explanation for this that has nothing to do with me?

9. **Control Fallacies.** There are two types of control fallacies: external and internal. In external control, you feel helpless and believe that control of your life rests in the hands of others, including your emotional state. An example of an external control fallacy is, *I want to be a good employee and have a good attitude, but I can't have a good attitude in my office environment.*

In internal control fallacies, you believe that you are responsible for everything and are in control of things that are truly beyond your control. The moods of others are a great example. People who use the internal control fallacy believe that it is their fault when others are in bad moods.

Internal Control Example: Mary feels responsible for her husband always being irritated when he gets home from work and believes she should have control over how he feels. This leads her to putting so much energy into every interaction with him that her own emotional exhaustion and self-blame leads to her using food to feel better.

External Control Example: I can never be successful with my diet as long as I have to work somewhere that makes sweet foods available during meetings.

Challenge Questions:

- What am I trying to control that is really out of my control?

- How can I begin to let go of that?

- Where do I believe that things are out of my control, but are actually where I can take more control and positively impact my life?

- How can I do a better job of "letting go"?

10. **Fallacy of Fairness.** This cognitive distortion makes you believe life should be fair. When it's not, you have negative feelings that allow you to reinforce your negative core beliefs about yourself. These in turn produce emotions that eventually cause the self-sabotaging behavior that reinforces those negative core beliefs.

At the conscious level, when you, for example, believe it is not fair that others find it easy to keep weight off, an emotional state is produced that does not help you reach your weight loss goals. However, at the subconscious level, if you believe that life should be fair and people get what they deserve, your inability to lose weight just proves your negative core beliefs about yourself to be true.

Example: You believe that it is not fair that others are able to lose weight easier than you or seem to be born with the right genetics that keeps them from having to struggle. This puts you in a non-resourceful emotional state while also confirming to you that if life is fair, you must not deserve to be thin.

Challenge Questions:

- Are there areas other than weight where someone would look at me and say that I am the one that has an unfair advantage?

- In what ways am I viewing this only through the eyes of this one issue?

- What happens when I look at all of my skills and abilities and those of others as a whole?

- How can my struggles eventually be a gift to me and others by overcoming them? (My own life is far better for having been overweight and having overcome it, than if I had been fit my whole life. The lessons I have learned and the skills I have developed as a result have not only made my life better in every area but have allowed me to help many others. What is the treasure in your struggle?)

11. **Blaming.** When you blame others, you make them responsible for your own feelings and actions. As you've learned through your understanding of the Inner Critic and now cognitive distortions, you are the one who, with your new skills and understandings, has control over how you feel. No one can make you feel any way other than how you allow them to make you feel. This is because it's not really them making you feel bad but what you make their words mean in your own head.

    Blaming others not only takes responsibility away from you, it also disempowers you. If others are responsible for your problems or bad feelings, then by inference, you do not have the ability to control those things yourself and improve your life.

    Example: Blaming others for tempting you to eat or putting you in the emotional states that cause you to not make healthy food choices or not exercise.

    Challenge Questions:

    - How can I accept more responsibility for this situation or plan in advance for similar situations to keep them from happening again?

- Regardless of how I feel, does blaming others help me reach my goals, or does blaming others keep me stuck by framing me as powerless?

12. **Shoulds.** Any time you use the word "should," you imply a judgment about the way you believe something ought to be. That judgment is based on your own internal rules, usually interjected from childhood, about how the world should operate. Every time you tell yourself that you should do something, you judge yourself negatively.

Judgment makes people feel bad and is a very ineffective motivation strategy. Take note of how you use the word "should" because it can point the way to understanding your internal rules. Those internal rules may be in conflict with achieving the feelings required to motivate you to stay with your weight loss goals.

Take note of the next time you use the word "should" about some behavior you are not doing or some way that you believe you are deficient. Notice your emotional state; most likely you will feel less motivated to do whatever you "should do."

Examples: I shouldn't be fat. I shouldn't be lazy. I should be thinner. I should work out more.

Challenge Questions:

- Who says I should?

- Where does this belief come from?

- Is this a belief I want in my life?

- What would happen if I didn't?

- Would I be more inclined to do and enjoy this if I wanted to do it instead of feeling like I should?

- How can I let go of the "should" and bring more joy to doing this?

13. **Emotional Reasoning.** Emotional reasoning occurs when you filter your experience through your current emotional state, and you assume that how you feel is how things are. For example, if you feel stupid then you must be stupid. If you feel fat or unattractive then it must be true. When you use emotional reasoning, you believe your emotions over facts or other evidence. *I feel it, so it must be true* characterizes this distortion.

   Example: You may not have lost the weight that you wanted to this week, so you feel defeated. Because of this emotional state, you believe it's impossible for you to reach your final goal weight and you give up and start eating whatever you can find. In reality, outside of how you were feeling in that moment, you'd done exceptionally well on your diet overall and had you not given up you would've succeeded.

   Challenge Questions:

   - Regardless of how I feel now, what evidence do I have that this is true?

   - Can I find evidence that it is not true?

   - Does it serve me to believe this is true, or would I be better off if I acted from a space of knowing it is not true until my feelings catch up with the truth?

14. **Global Labeling.** Global labeling is when you take a limited amount of experiences, and then apply them at a level that goes far beyond the scope of what those experiences actually suggest. For example, you may fail a test at school, and at the same time you fail to get a promotion at work. From these two events you decide you are a complete loser, despite excelling in several other areas of your life.

Example: The most common way people who suffer from chronic weight issues use this cognitive distortion is when they judge their entire lives based on their weight. *I'm fat, therefore I'm unattractive; I'm overweight, so I'm a complete loser.*

Challenge Questions:

- Is this true all the time in all situations?

- In what situations is this not true?

- Based on knowing that this is not true all the time, what is the actual truth?

- How can I be more open minded about this until I look at all of the evidence?

15. **Heaven's Reward Fallacy.** In this cognitive distortion, you believe you will eventually be rewarded for your suffering. Later in this book, you will learn about what is called secondary gains, which are benefits you subconsciously believe you will get from not doing what you consciously want to do. Those who use this cognitive distortion often self-sabotage themselves in many areas of their lives, believing that there is nobility or an eventual payoff to their suffering.

    Example: The diabetic or heart patient that continues to eat unhealthy and be obese because they subconsciously believe that they are a better person for suffering.

    Challenge Questions:

    - Why do I believe that there is nobility in suffering?

    - Do I know good people that I admire who do not suffer?

    - What do I get out of preserving this belief?

    - How could my life be better if I changed this belief?

The Inner Critic uses all of these cognitive distortions to make what it says sound true, yet when these cognitive distortions are challenged, you will find they quickly fall apart and lose their power.

EXERCISE: YOUR INNER CRITIC ON TRIAL

For the next step in the process, go through all of the Inner Critic statements that you accumulated in the last exercise and see how many cognitive distortions you can find. Apply the appropriate challenge questions and see how quickly these cognitive distortions and the Inner Critic lose power over you.

If you have the *Fat to Fearless*® Success Guide and Workbook, then you will see under each of the Inner Critic statements is space to write the cognitive distortions you find within each statement, as well as a place to write the challenge questions and your answers. If you do not have the workbook, do this on a separate sheet of paper. Do this exercise right now.

After you've completed this exercise, answer the following questions:

1. After challenging the cognitive distortions within the Inner Critic's statements, how did it affect the level of power, impact, and truth that the statement seemed to previously have?

2. Can you see how these cognitive distortions trick you into believing the Inner Critic by presenting statements with distorted, generalized, or deleted information?

3. If you were to train yourself constantly to catch Inner Critical Statements when they occur and immediately challenge any cognitive distortions, what impact do you think that would have on your overall emotional state? How do you believe that your changed emotional state would impact your ability to stay with a healthy eating plan?

After completing this exercise, you now understand how the Inner Critic uses cognitive distortions to make lies about you seem true and impact your emotional state and beliefs about yourself. You have also learned how you can challenge those cognitive distortions and begin to disempower the Inner Critic.

Your job now is to do this all the time until it becomes so automatic that the Inner Critic begins to change. This section is about conscious change, which means making conscious effort, and these processes will change your life. But they do require you to work at them.

For the next month, carry your notebook or workbook with you and begin immediately catching any Inner Critical statement. Then analyze them for cognitive distortions, challenge any that you find, and watch them lose their power.

It can also be helpful to listen to how others talk in conversation and try to find cognitive distortions in their speech. As you do this, try to find how these cognitive distortions may be affecting your behavior, decisions, and emotions.

In the next exercise, you're going to learn to use the power of humor to tame the Inner Critic even more.

Use Humor and Affirmations Against the Inner Critic

In the first exercise in this chapter, you not only logged exactly what your Inner Critic was saying to you, but how it was saying it as well. Specifically, you learned about submodalities and recorded them in your workbook. Remember submodalities, as it specifically applies to this internal voice, are things like how loud it is, pitch, tempo, the emotional quality of the voice, etc. This wasn't the first time that you were exposed to submodalities; you also used them with your New Body Movie Trailer.

You had a chance to see how powerful changing submodalities (details of how you represent things to yourself) can be when you changed the visual submodalities in your New Body Movie Trailer. Now you will use the same technique to reduce the power of the Inner Critic.

1. In previous exercises, you determined all of the audio submodalities of the Inner Critic. You discerned things like:

   a. How loud it is

   b. The tone

   c. Emotionally sounding attributes

   d. The direction it's coming from

   e. Tempo and speed

   Review these submodalities now. You may have all of those listed above, or just a few, or some not on the list.

2. In this step, you want to change the submodalities of the voice until it no longer has a negative effect. In fact, you want to change it to something that is humorous and hard to take seriously. Try doing some of these:

   a. Change the Inner Critic to Donald Duck's voice or some other funny cartoon character. Any time you catch the Inner Critic talking to you, and at this point you're becoming very good at spotting it, *immediately* change it to this funny voice. If you do this often enough it will become automatic.

   b. Change the direction that the voice is coming from. Many people find that the Inner Critic seems to boom down from above or behind them. Change the Inner Critic's voice to come from below, as if it is small and beneath you.

   c. Reduce the volume of the Inner Critic, so that it not only sounds like a funny cartoon voice and it is coming from below, but that—as it continues to talk—it becomes quieter and quieter until it disappears entirely.

3. Create a funny visual image of the Inner Critic, some type of caricature that underscores how little power it has. Some people actually use the image of Donald Duck while others create an image that for whatever reason denotes powerlessness to them. Soon you will think of the Inner Critic as this caricature and what it represents as small and powerless, and so in time it shall actually become.

Another reframe that will disempower the Inner Critic is to realize that, while sounding like an adult, it is actually as much a child as the Inner Child you will soon be learning more about. The Inner Critic was created when you were a child and therefore is nothing more than a child's interpretation of an adult authority voice. Often clients find that seeing the Inner Critic as a spoiled child trying to act like an adult by asserting its non-existent authority brings further humor and disempowerment to it while making it easier to dismiss its criticisms.

Everything we are doing together works by repetition, and while this may sound silly, you will find that after a month of constantly and consciously doing this every time you hear the Inner Critic it will begin to become automatic, and it will lose even more of its power.

This exercise is one that you really must try to see how effective it can be! When just reading it, you can't truly appreciate how quickly it can create change. Combining humor with reversing cognitive distortions, if done persistently and with repetition, will have your Inner Critic ready to surrender!

SUMMARY

Key Points

- Your Inner Critic works to preserve your negative core beliefs and seems to be a part of you. This negative voice in your head seems to arise spontaneously with little choice on your part.

- Transforming the Inner Critic into a healthier voice is both a conscious and a subconscious process.

- Listening to your *Fat to Fearless*® Hypnotherapy Audio Sessions while also using your affirmations with their delivery system works at the subconscious level to begin to change the Inner Critic.

- The conscious process of changing the Inner Critic is learning to identify it when you hear it and separate it from the real you while also learning to disarm it by recognizing and reversing its cognitive distortions and applying humor and submodality changes.

- Cognitive distortions are ways that your mind convinces you that something is true, that actually is not, by linguistically distorting your perception.

- Any time you hear the word "should" in your internal dialogue, followed by a bad feeling or a feeling of not "living up to expectations" you are most likely hearing the Inner Critic speak.

- The Inner Critic fuels the Symptom Cycle, which tells us that the way you feel about being overweight is the indirect cause of the behaviors that keep you overweight. Eating to feel better is the perfect example.

- Keeping an Inner Critic Journal for a week is a great way to learn to identify this internal negative voice and separate it from the "real you."

- Once you become conscious of cognitive distortions and challenge them with questions that reveal the truth, they quickly lose their power.

- Using humor is another way of disempowering the Inner Critic. By changing its voice to one that is hard to take seriously as well as associating a funny or non-threatening image with it, the Inner Critic loses even more of its ability to negatively affect you.

- In time, if done with enough repetition, all of these consciously applied techniques of disempowering the Inner Critic will become unconscious and automatic.

What This Has To Do With Weight Loss

Behind every emotional food binge and diet that's dishearteningly abandoned, you will find the negative voice of the Inner Critic. Shaking the control this voice has over you is not only critical to your long-term weight loss success and enabling you to transform your core beliefs but is also critical to stopping the negative feelings in the moments that lead to emotional eating.

You Are Ready To Move On When . . .

- You are easily able to identify the voice of the Inner Critic and separate it from the true you.

- You have learned to automatically challenge what the Inner Critic says by listening for cognitive distortions and applying the appropriate challenge questions.

  There is a dramatic decrease in the Inner Critic's ability to negatively impact you through a combination of challenging its cognitive distortions as well as changing the quality of the voice and associating an image with it that makes it hard to take seriously if not outright funny.

- You have watched the tutorial video for this chapter (if you have the full *Fat to Fearless*® program).

- You have completed the exercises for this chapter in the Success Guide and Workbook (if you have the full *Fat to Fearless*® program).

- You are listening to you Hypnotherapy Audio Sessions according to their included instructions (if you have the full *Fat to Fearless*® program).

CHAPTER 16

REPROGRAM THE R.A.S.

A s you learned previously, one of the ways of influencing the subconscious mind is through repetition. If the conscious mind is insistent enough, eventually the subconscious begins to listen. The challenge is that the conscious mind has trouble being persistent when it is fighting the emotions generated by the subconscious, the R.A.S filtering out information that contradicts our existing beliefs, and the Inner Critic and its cognitive distortions working against us. In the midst of this, it is hard to remember all of the circumstances that life has given us to prove that we are valuable and worthwhile and that we deserve to have the body we want. This is why you are going to create an evidence journal.

As you've already learned, the Reticular Activating System tends to only bring to conscious awareness information that is either critical to our immediate survival (the speeding car at the intersection we see out of the corner of our eye) or information that's consistent with our already existing core beliefs (the conversation in the corner of the room that when we overhear the word "fat" we mind-read and assume must be about us).

When you change your core beliefs, you automatically give the R.A.S. new programming instructions to search for information that's consistent with those new beliefs. Therefore, all of the work that you are currently doing and have done so far is working to subconsciously reprogram the R.A.S. to help you reach your weight loss goals by installing new and supportive core beliefs. An evidence journal is a way of using your conscious mind to begin training your R.A.S. to subconsciously seek out proof in your environment that supports your new beliefs and healthy weight loss goals.

I developed the evidence journal several years ago in response to my own realization that when I was feeling bad about myself and my self-esteem was low, I could not remember the positive experiences that contradicted what I was feeling bad about. I had the vague awareness that they had happened, but couldn't specifically remember them well enough to use them to feel better.

The specific instance that I remember most vividly was when I was really down on myself after I believed I had been rejected by a woman I was interested in. Immediately, because of my past childhood programming and from being an overweight child, my core beliefs that I was unattractive and undesirable took center stage in my mind. I felt incredibly unworthy and unattractive, even though I knew that I had recently been asked out by several attractive women.

Before believing that I had been rejected by this woman, I had just been wondering why so many women seemed to be flirting with me, complimenting me, and asking me out recently. Yet when I was feeling bad about myself from this one instance, I literally could not remember the specifics of a single instance of those previous encounters that confirmed my desirability even though I knew intellectually it had happened several times in the prior weeks. My subconscious was blocking, or at least making it hard to remember, those memories that conflicted with my core beliefs of being unattractive and undesirable. This was when I decided to keep an evidence journal.

An evidence journal is an ongoing list of experiences that contradict your negative core beliefs. It's evidence of the truth.

I started by listing in my journal every time a woman showed interest in me, went out of her way to compliment me, or asked me out. From then on, whenever I had an experience that made me feel those old beliefs of being undesirable, I reached for my evidence journal and consciously reviewed all of the proof to the contrary. Within minutes my feelings would change. Over a period of time—through repetition—this had an impact on these subconscious beliefs. What I didn't realize at the time was the impact it was having on my R.A.S., and how that was contributing to the changing beliefs. Let's do a quick experiment.

Take a look around the room and tell me how many things you can see in your field of vision that are blue. How many did you find? Without looking again, how many objects that were in your field of vision were brown? Other than a few objects that you already know from memory that are brown and in the room, like a couch for example, you probably do not know because you and your R.A.S. were looking for things colored blue.

In addition to the subconscious filtering process of the R.A.S, you also use it consciously. As you know, anything you do consciously with enough repetition will eventually pass to the subconscious mind and become an automated process. If every time you walked into a room you searched for objects that were blue, you would eventually start doing it without even thinking about it. You can use the same principle with your evidence journal to consciously program your R.A.S. to automatically find evidence every day that supports your new positive beliefs.

Changing people's minds—as well as their beliefs, patterns, and habits—is based on what is called a threshold response. A threshold response is a change that occurs based on the cumulative level of input reaching the level needed to create a change. In other words, the tipping point. It also has a relationship to how long or short a period in which this input occurs. The greater the input in the shorter the time period, the quicker change occurs.

An evidence journal reprograms your R.A.S. so it contradicts your old beliefs. Eventually your subconscious reaches the threshold response necessary for your beliefs to change. This was exactly how it worked for me.

I accumulated so much evidence that contradicted my negative core beliefs that it became impossible to convince myself that I was completely undesirable to women. If someone I was interested in didn't reciprocate, I could open my evidence journal and read page after page of experiences that showed that many women were interested in me.

After that, I would no longer be able to tell myself the cognitively distorted lie that I was undesirable. Instead, I told myself the truth: *I am more than good enough; I just wasn't this woman's type. I know that I will meet the right person.* While rejection is never very pleasant, it stings much less when viewed though the eyes of truth.

Now let's apply this same process to you.

EXERCISE: EVIDENCE JOURNAL

1. Review the top five new core beliefs you are programming yourself with and the top five negative core beliefs you want to change.

2. Think of as many past experiences as possible that show your positive core beliefs are true and the old negative core beliefs are false. Log these experiences in your evidence journal. It's okay if you can't find many; it just means your R.A.S. with its old programming did not pick up on them and not that they didn't happen.

Here are some examples:

If your old core belief is that you are not good enough, remember times you got promotions, had exceptional grades in school, or received compliments that indicated that you are more than good enough.

If your old core belief is that you are ugly or unattractive, remember times you were asked out or complimented by friends, family, or a significant other, or when someone obviously noticed you out in public.

If your old core belief is that you are a loser, remember every accomplishment—large and small.

If you believe you can't lose weight, remember every time you managed to successfully lose weight in the past regardless of how long it stayed off.

If you believe that you were not born with the right genetics to lose weight and keep it off, remember times that you either read or heard about people who felt the same way but were successful.

Once you are done with this, you will have some initial entries in your evidence journal. You can also collect the experiences of role models and others you can relate to whose achievements contradict your negative beliefs.

3. Now the fun part begins. Your job now is to go on a daily scavenger hunt for information and experiences that prove your old core beliefs are false and that your new ones are true. To keep your R.A.S. focused on this new information, review what has transpired in your day every two to three hours, and then focus again on the task of consciously looking for positive core belief evidence. The more you find, the closer you get to the threshold response necessary to shift your old core beliefs to new ones. You will also reprogram your R.A.S. so that finding, noticing, and experiencing positive things that reinforce your new desirable beliefs becomes automatic.

4. Any time you feel bad and are tempted to believe that those old beliefs are true, review your evidence journal and realize they definitely are not true. If you find

yourself doubting the evidence journal, then you must also be hearing the voice of the Inner Critic. Immediately apply all that you have learned in the prior sections to defeat your Inner Critic, and then re-examine your evidence journal without interference.

SUMMARY

Key Points

- Reprogramming your Reticular Activating System (R.A.S.) to search for new information that confirms your new healthier beliefs is essential to long-term weight loss success.

- All of the work you are doing in the *Fat to Fearless*® program to change your core beliefs is also changing what information your R.A.S. searches for in your environment and brings to your conscious awareness.

- In addition to the subconscious changes that are taking place that are redirecting your R.A.S.' focus, you can also use your conscious mind to program your R.A.S. to search for evidence that your new weight-loss-supporting beliefs are true. Eventually, this will become automatic.

- An evidence journal enables you to always have access to proof that the new beliefs you are installing are true, while also reprogramming your R.A.S. to search for new experiences that confirm that truth.

What This Has To Do With Weight Loss

Reprogramming the R.A.S. will allow you to notice and become aware of experiences and information that supports both your intellectual need to know you're on the right track as well as supports you in maintaining a healthy emotional state during the weight loss process.

You Are Ready To Move To The Next Chapter When . . .

- You have watched the tutorial video for this chapter (if you have the full *Fat to Fearless*® program).

- You have completed the exercises for this chapter in the Success Guide and Workbook (if you have the full *Fat to Fearless*® program).

PART V

EATING AND YOUR EMOTIONS

CHAPTER 17

EMOTIONAL SELF-SOOTHING

You now understand that negative emotions are the result of experiencing life through the filter of negative core beliefs. You know that changing those core beliefs into life-affirming positive beliefs results in new positive emotions as well.

When you change your core beliefs to positive ones you create new positive filters for life and your emotions also transform into positive emotions that you no longer need to soothe through food.

One of the challenges with weight loss is how long it takes to change these beliefs, and then the lag time for your emotions to change in relationship to how easy it is to quickly gain weight. If you worked through the exercises in the last sections, you are well on your way to having new positive core beliefs that support you to lose weight now. (If you didn't, I strongly suggest that you go back and work through the exercises.) Within a month you will begin to feel and experience life differently. Unfortunately, the emotions that make you want to eat to feel better tend to happen every day and even with a program like *Fat to Fearless*® that quickly creates change at the core belief level, that often isn't fast enough to stop emotional eating in the moment.

If you focus solely on core belief change alone it may take a full 90 days to see the type of significant change in your core beliefs that leads to a noticeable reduction in negative emotions, which in turn keeps you from turning to food to feel better. Remember that many of these emotions are habitual with well-developed neural pathways that make it easy for your brain to head down those negative paths. But it's not just these negative emotional responses that have well-developed neural pathways, but the unhealthy eating behaviors that are paired with these emotions as well. You can see why it is important to have a tool to directly address emotional self-soothing through food—in the now—while your new positive core beliefs are taking hold and beginning to change your thoughts, feelings, and habits for the future.

Emotional self-soothing is perhaps the one cause of overeating that is most easily recognized and understood by everyone with a weight problem. Most people who struggle with eating issues know that most of the time when they eat they just want to feel better emotionally.

Food, especially most of the food that is bad for you, often feels like the first defense against emotions you don't want to experience. That is why they are called comfort foods. When I look back at my own struggles with food I can tell you I rarely overate or ate too much of the wrong foods out of hunger. Instead, it was out of a deeper need to feel better emotionally in that moment.

The need to self-soothe with food can be incredibly strong. The most dramatic instance of this that I can remember in my own life was during the same period of time I mentioned in the introduction to this book, just a few weeks out from a video shoot in which I needed to look my best.

I remember going to the local grocery store with the thought of having a "cheat meal" of sushi. I was proud that I had chosen something to cheat with that was actually quite healthy given my normal "cheat food" choices. I walked into that store, never imagining that I would walk out with my weight loss goal's sugary doom.

On my way to pick up the sushi, I passed through the bakery where the bright icing of the cupcakes caught my eye. My first mistake was stopping to look, and it was all downhill from there. The first step is often the easiest, and is always the one that eventually leads to the final step.

Deciding to stop and look at the cupcakes, as innocent as that may have seemed, led to a three-hour binge of cookies, cupcakes, and ice cream. I can remember holding the cupcakes up to my face wishing that I could taste them through the plastic. I knew I had a real problem when I actually began considering how I could get my finger inside just to taste them.

The interesting thing about that moment where I thought about how I could get my finger inside the package was the absurdity of it. I was an intelligent, mature, successful adult. In my right mind I would never consider trying to covertly stick my finger into a sealed box of cupcakes I did not intend to buy, anymore than I would shoplift them.

But the voice that had that thought didn't arise from my conscious thoughts, but came directly out of my subconscious. For a moment I felt possessed by some "other me" buried deep inside, a me that did not feel good and desperately wanted to use those cupcakes to feel better.

With my training and experience as a Subconscious Behaviorist, once this part of me gave up control, several hours and unimaginable amounts of sugar later, I understood what had happened and what the next step in my healing journey needed to be to keep this from happening again.

If any of this sounds familiar to you, then the coming pages and exercises will give you the tools you need to change this behavior, and perhaps more importantly, to heal that part of you that reaches for food to alleviate its pain.

You are already familiar with one voice in your head, the Inner Critic. Every time you tell yourself you are fat or stupid, or criticize yourself in a way that makes you feel bad, you are hearing the Inner Critic speak. You have also learned how to disempower this negative voice so that it has less influence in your life.

The voice with which you may not be as familiar is the one that emotionally responds to those criticisms, because it often speaks with feelings rather than with words. You are familiar with these emotions and the negative behaviors they lead to. This other part of you is the one that is actually crying out for the food in order to feel better because it is the part of you that is actually hurting. It is time for you to learn about your Inner Child.

There are several ways to heal painful emotions, and they are all effective to some degree. However, the most effective model is one where you label your thoughts and feelings in a way that allows you to objectively understand them, and then heal the source of these unpleasant feelings.

You experienced the power of this when you learned to label the thoughts of the Inner Critic and confront them directly. Likewise, understanding your emotional nature and why it drives you to self-sabotage is the fastest path to eliminating emotional self-soothing. In many psychological models, this emotional nature is referred to as the Inner Child. Learning about the Inner Child gives you a framework for understanding the nature of the emotions you try to soothe with food, as well as where they originated. It will also give you a set of tools to stop emotional eating while you are waiting for your day-to-day feelings to catch up with the new healthier core beliefs you are creating.

If you suffer from chronic sadness, low self-esteem, feelings of emptiness, or any other type of ongoing negative emotions, somewhere inside of you is a wounded child that needs you to rescue them so they can stop using food to feel better about themselves.

One of the reasons this may not be easy for you to accept is because you have not talked to this child inside of you, your Inner Child, in a long time. You may be disconnected from it, and thus disconnected from understanding your emotions. This child inside may also feel that you have abandoned them. They might distrust you, your conscious mind, and your intentions as you begin to communicate with him or her. Reclaiming and healing this Inner Child may not be an easy task, but it is one with huge rewards.

You are going to learn to speak the language of the Inner Child in a way allows you to hear it, understand it, and help it to heal so that it no longer craves food to feel better.

EXERCISE: GLIMPSING YOUR INNER CHILD

Step 1
Because of the term being liberally and often incorrectly used in pop psychology, people often have negative associations with the term "Inner Child." In the space provided in your Success Guide and Workbook, list any thoughts or preconceptions you may have about the concept of an Inner Child that may interfere with you now being open to doing this work.

After doing so, make a commitment to suspend these preconceived ideas that may possibly act as blocks to the effectiveness of the Inner Child work you are now going to do. Also, remember if it makes it easier, you can just think of your Inner Child as your "emotional self."

Step 2
Everyone begins this journey with a certain amount of existing awareness of their childlike self. In the blanks provided in your Success Guide and Workbook list times in your life, either present of past, in which you have come in contact with your Inner Child.

Perhaps these are times you have found yourself throwing a tantrum, or enjoying the pure joy of something wonderfully simple, or allowed yourself a selfish moment, or simply felt the desire to be held by someone that loved you. While you may not realize it now, every time you have reached for food to feel better, you were also having an Inner Child experience.

SUMMARY

Key Points

- Negative emotions are the result of experiencing life through the filter of negative core beliefs.

- When you change your core beliefs to positive ones your emotions also transform into positive emotions that you no longer need to soothe through food.

- One of the challenges with losing weight is the lag time between your beliefs changing and the time it takes to experience that emotionally. While, with a program like *Fat to Fearless®* it will happen quickly, it often isn't fast enough to stop you from emotionally eating on a day-to-day basis as you go through the process.

- While changing your core beliefs addresses the root cause of emotional eating, it's also important to have a tool to deal directly with the emotional symptoms on a day-to-day basis as you are going through the program.

- Allowing yourself to consider eating foods that go against your weight loss plan, or even giving yourself mental permission to imagine them, is usually what begins the process of an emotional eating episode.

- The part of you that is crying out for food to feel better is the Inner Child. You can think of it as your "emotional self."

- Using the model of labeling your emotional self as your Inner Child will give you the path and the tools to deal directly with this needy emotional voice in the same way labeling the Inner Critic allowed us to deal with the negative voice in your head.

What This Has To Do With Weight Loss

The biggest reason stated for long-term weight loss failure is emotional eating. It's difficult to deal with something in a way to change it unless we can objectively look at it. Our emotions are the same way. The Inner Child model gives us a way to separate from our emotions to enable us to apply a variety of tools to transform those wounded emotions and heal early childhood damage before ultimately reintegrating this child back into ourselves, allowing us to become a more complete whole.

The Inner Child model of healing is one of the most powerful ways of transforming the emotions that drive you to eat in the moment into more positive emotions that support you in losing weight.

You Are Ready To Move To The Next Chapter When . . .

- You have made a decision to embrace the Inner Child model of emotional healing. For some who don't fully understand this model the concept of a "child" living in your subconscious is difficult to accept. If this is you, feel free to think of it as just your "emotional self." Labeling this part of yourself is integral to your ability to separate from it so you can eventually heal it and fully integrate it back into yourself as a whole.

- You have watched the tutorial video for this chapter (if you have the full *Fat to Fearless*® program).

- You have completed the exercises for this chapter in the Success Guide and Workbook (if you have the full *Fat to Fearless*® program).

CHAPTER 18

UNDERSTANDING THE INNER CHILD

Most of us are familiar with the term "Inner Child" from popular culture and pop psychology, but few know exactly what it is and how it came to be.

Think of the Inner Child as your original and true self. It was who you were before life ever gave you the idea that you should be anyone else. Your Inner Child is the emotional part of you that plays a large role in your emotional self-soothing behaviors as well as in other ways that keep you from reaching your weight loss goals.

To understand this and to begin to change it, it is important to understand how the Inner Child is formed as well as what other parts of your psyche may be interacting with your Inner Child to keep you from the change you want.

Have you ever found yourself arguing with yourself? While you have probably never really thought much about it, it may often seem like there are parts of yourself that war with each other. In the therapy world, these parts are sometimes referred to as subpersonalities.

Subpersonalities are not multiple personalities or anything abnormal; they are actually just different perspectives or points of view that form around different sets of experiences, motivations, and often conflicting beliefs. This can happen around almost anything.

For example, there might be a part of you that doesn't want to quit your job because you like the perceived financial security, but there might be another part of you that dreams of starting your own business and believes that you should. The conflict you have around this is an internal argument between these parts.

Sometimes you have "parts conflicts" around larger issues, such as the part of you that might want to stay with your spouse and the part of you that might want to leave. Sometimes you have "parts conflicts" around small issues, such as the part that likes corn chips and the part that likes potato chips. Normally this last one isn't a problem unless they decide to fight it out in the grocery store aisle.

These types of parts are always being changed, created, and recreated within us based on new experiences, perspectives, and ideas. There are, however, three parts of us that tend to be relatively constant and form a core part of our psyche. Without intervention, they may not change much throughout our entire lives. These three parts are often referred to as our primary ego states and consist of our Inner Child, the Inner Critic, and our adult self.

Let us look at how these three ego states interact and how that pertains to the negative emotions that often cause you to self-sabotage your weight loss goals.

The Inner Child is who you are when you are born. Often called "the original self," the Inner Child is all you know of who you are in the very early stages of life.

When you are first born, you are free of the judgments of others, have no concern for rules (because you have no idea what they are anyway), and are able to fully express yourself in whatever way you see fit as you begin to explore this exciting new world you have unexpectedly found yourself in.

This state of bliss does not last very long. You are born into a social system, culture, and family that has expectations about who, how, and what you are supposed to be, do, and become. You start realizing this at a very early age.

As you have already learned, it is during this period of early socialization that the Inner Critic begins to form to keep the child safe. It helps the child conform to its community by regulating behavior with a list of "shoulds" and expectations. Since it's designed to keep you in line and make sure you conform, so as not to get kicked out of your family or social unit (the tribe), it is typically a negative voice that motivates with a stick instead of a carrot.

As you age and grow older, this original self does not go away nor does its childlike nature. Instead, the Inner Critic often suppresses the Inner Child through criticism of its childlike nature, which the Inner Critic often judges as being in conflict with the expectations to which it is trying to force you to conform.

Without this criticism, the Inner Child would be able to go through a healthy maturation process that would enable it to eventually become integrated into your psyche resulting in a more psychologically complete and balanced person. Instead, because of the harsh judgments of the Inner Critic, the Inner Child often becomes internalized, buried, suppressed, and often forgotten by your adult self.

As you've learned, things of which you are not aware of that are in the subconscious often have even more power because of their hidden nature. Therefore, though often forgotten, the Inner Child continues to play a major role in influencing your life. Since the Inner Child is essentially your "emotional self," it does this by creating feelings that motivate your behavior.

Childhood emotional wounds are carried by the Inner Child, which you feel in the form of negative emotions. Most people, without the awareness of what is truly going on within themselves, try to alleviate these negative emotions through things outside of themselves, such as food, sex, drugs, shopping, or overworking.

Until you stop looking outside of yourself for relief and instead turn inside and begin to communicate with this Inner Child and understand what it needs to heal, you will never find peace. You need to love yourself and your Inner Child in a way that does not require seeking satisfaction with the things that ultimately take you further away from your goals.

Healing this wounded child inside of you begins with understanding its language. The Inner Child speaks, sometimes with words, but more often with emotions. It speaks with visceral gut feelings. Every time you feel lonely, sad, or hopeless—in that moment before reaching out for food, you experience what that Inner Child is feeling. These are moments that provide an opportunity to connect with yourself at a deeper level and begin the process of changing and healing.

Instead, because you do not realize this is an opportunity to make contact with and begin to heal this part of yourself, you try to make the feeling go away any way you can. For the chronically overweight, food is usually the first "medicine" that is turned to during these emotional moments. However counterintuitive it may seem, you now want to tune into these negative feelings and use them as an opportunity to communicate with yourself at a deeper level. Sit with them, go inside them, and begin listening for that disconnected little boy or girl inside of you that desperately wants to feel better.

Although the child speaks through emotion, sometimes it gives words to those emotions. When you hear yourself saying one of the following phrases during a time you are feeling "bad" it is usually the Inner Child speaking:

> *I want...*
>
> *It's not fair...*
>
> Give me...

When you find yourself saying statements like these when you are feeling strong emotion, it is a great opportunity to check in and get a sense of the feelings behind them and the part of you from which they originate. You typically go through life feeling what you feel, and when that feeling is unpleasant, you either try to figure out why you feel that or you find something outside yourself to feel better. Both of these are strategies to avoid dealing with the actual feelings themselves. Every time you feel these negative emotions and ignore them or try to intellectualize them by "figuring it out," you ignore your Inner Child's pain, sending it a message that only ends up making things worse.

Imagine that you had a real child that was crying. You would not simply ignore this child or try to distract yourself, would you? You also wouldn't try to figure out why your child was upset before soothing it would you? Yet that is exactly what your adult self does every time you avoid dealing with the feelings of your Inner Child.

Worse, when you do this you tell your Inner Child that you do not care about it or its feelings, which only causes the feelings to come back stronger because the source of these feelings is the child's negative beliefs that are then reinforced through your messages of neglect.

The negative core beliefs that you are overcoming and changing are predominately the beliefs of your Inner Child. While you are changing this child's beliefs through all of the work you are now doing, the current emotional state of the child while your doing this can't be ignored. If it is, the child will continue to reach out for food to feel better and sabotage all of the other efforts you are making toward healing yourself and reprogramming your subconscious mind for weight loss success.

To understand what specifically happens when you self-soothe through food, you need to learn more about how the psyche evolves and to identify these different parts of yourself. Emotional difficulties often arise when the Inner Critic and Inner Child conflict. When this happens, a third part of your psyche arises to mediate, your adult self.

Your Inner Critic is almost always rooted in judgment, and it can be identified because it usually tells you that you are a direct reflection of your negative core beliefs. It frequently points out your deficiencies and often uses the word "should" to cement that judgment. It will say things like:

You should've known better. You're such an idiot!

Only you could be so stupid to do that again!

You should've done better. I can't believe you didn't see this coming!

If you were prettier, they would've picked you.

Your Inner Child, however, usually comes from a place of more visceral emotional need and frequently uses the words "need," "want," or other language you would expect the child to use. The Inner Child often says things like:

I want it.

I need it.

It isn't fair.

If only...

Your adult self is your logical, rational mind, the part you most often think with and identify as "you." Another way of looking at it is that your adult self is your conscious mind. While the other two voices, the Inner Critic and the Inner Child, seem to spontaneously arise on their own and live in your subconscious, you typically identify yourself consciously with your adult self.

It can sometimes be difficult to tell between the voice of the Inner Critic and your adult self because they may at times have similar messages. Typically, if you are hearing the language of the Inner Critic ("shoulds", self-blame, etc.) as well as experiencing negative emotions about yourself, it is the Inner Critic.

Let's say that in the past you have put yourself in difficult financial situations because of irresponsible spending, yet have been working on this issue to have a healthier perspective and behaviors around money. While the message may be the same (don't spend irresponsibly), the way it is delivered will be different. For example:

Inner Critic: "You know you shouldn't buy that because you always overspend and end up putting yourself in a bad financial spot. Why do you always do this to yourself? Why do you never learn?"

Adult Self: "I do want this now, but if I wait until the end of the month and then reassess my finances after paying my bills and seeing if I get the raise in pay I'm expecting, I can buy it without creating additional financial stress for myself."

As you can see, your adult self uses reason and logic without needing to resort to self-condemnation.

The way these ego states interact with each other, especially the Inner Critic and Inner Child, is the primary cause of the feelings that result in self-soothing through food. The Inner Critic develops simultaneously with your negative core beliefs and is essentially the henchman of these beliefs and seeks to preserve them with its negative and judging messages. These messages create a negative emotional reaction within your Inner Child that makes you want to turn to food for comfort.

When the Inner Critic says something that makes you feel bad, it is your Inner Child (your emotional self) that is having the emotional reaction that you're feeling. When the Inner Critic says, *I'm too ugly to think he would want to go out with me*, or *I should've known I couldn't keep the weight off, I just need to accept that I'm fat*, it is the Inner Child that hears that message and feels its impact.

The Inner Child, the source of our most powerful emotions, is the one that feels those feelings of sadness, shame, hopelessness, fear, and loneliness. Those feelings cause us to reach for anything to make us feel better. For the chronically overweight, what you reach for first is food.

To stop self-soothing through food, the negative voice of the Inner Critic must be disempowered so that it has less of an emotional impact on the Inner Child, while the Inner Child is being healed and empowered, which in turn allows you to feel good enough that you do not need immediate gratification. Here are steps to achieve this.

1. **Transform Negative Core Beliefs.** When you change negative core beliefs to positive ones, you also change the nature of the Inner Critic while also healing the Inner Child. You are, and have been since the beginning of the *Fat to Fearless*® program, in the process of doing this now.

2. **Recognize and Disempower The Inner Critic.** While transforming your negative core beliefs, it helps to become conscious of the Inner Critic when you hear it and recognize that it is not part of your true self. Consciously deny what it is telling you and dissect its cognitive distortions that you previously learned about that makes its falsehoods seem believable.

   Replace the Inner Critic's negative talk with the affirmations that you created that support the healthier core beliefs you are developing. To do this, you must recognize this negative voice when you hear it. Up to this point in your life, you have failed to make that distinction and you thought it was actually you. But now, with the work you have done already, you can clearly identify the Inner Critic and disempower it with the tools and techniques you learned in the prior chapters.

3. **Empowering the Inner Child.** As important as it is to disempower the Inner Critic, it is equally important to empower and heal the Inner Child. Your Inner Child has been the source of endless emotional abuse at the hands of the Inner Critic for most of your life. It has sustained significant emotional damage. Your Inner Child needs to be reparented for you to reach your full potential, not only in reaching your weight loss goals, but to also be able to enjoy and maintain it once you do.

The first step to empowering the Inner Child is to open up dialogue with him or her so that you can begin to communicate in a healthy and productive way. In the following exercise you're going to learn to do exactly that.

EXERCISE: INNER CHILD JOURNAL

One of the best ways to communicate with your Inner Child and begin the process of healing it is what I call an Inner Child Journal. As you just learned, one of the reasons behind the emotions that cause you to use food to self-soothe, is the Inner Child feeling neglected, unheard, or uncared for. Just like a real child, when it feels bad it reaches for what will give it the most immediate relief, and without any thought of the consequences. If you suffer from long-term weight issues, this has probably been food.

In this exercise you will use a journal to connect with your Inner Child and further understand what it needs from you while reassuring your child that you care, you are there, and you are going to work to meet its needs.

1. Purchase a journal that allows for you to write on both sides of each sheet of paper.

2. Set aside a time each night and take 15 minutes to communicate with your Inner Child using the journal. Any time you feel upset is also a good time to communicate with the Inner Child because you are already feeling his or her emotions.

3. The first step is to tell your Inner Child that you love him/her, are there for him/her, and you want to meet their needs. It may also be a good idea to lovingly apologize to your Inner Child for any harm you may have done by ignoring its needs in the past. Then ask your Inner Child how it is feeling.

4. Once you ask the Inner Child how it is feeling, close your eyes, go within, and try to connect with what you are feeling at a deep level. Go beyond your surface thoughts and move into your body. We feel our emotions in our body, usually in the space beneath our chin and above our waist. Become aware of this area of your body and "drop down into it." Often you can get in touch with what you are feeling by finding it physically in your body. It is important to close your eyes during this step because it automatically produces a shift in your brainwave state that makes it easier to get in touch with your emotions.

5. Once you have found the emotion, associate into it and allow yourself to feel it fully and completely. Imagine that you are that Inner Child, that younger you that is having those feelings. Open your eyes and with your non-dominant hand (left hand for most of us) write in the journal as the Inner Child, feeling those feelings, and respond to your adult self's question about how you are feeling. You want to write on the side of the page that matches the hand you are using. (Again, left for most people.)

6. Come out of the feeling and back into your adult self, and respond to the Inner Child with your dominant hand on the side of the paper that matches that hand (right for most of us). As you continue to do this, you will have pages where on one side your Inner Child is speaking and on the other side your adult self is speaking. Switching hands is important because your dominant hand has very direct and well-developed neural pathways to your conscious adult self. Switching to the non-dominant hand makes it easier to bypass your conscious mind and speak from your subconscious.

7. After you have responded to the Inner Child, close your eyes, get back into the emotion and become the child again, and then respond back to the adult.

8. Continue to dialogue back and forth between your Inner Child and adult self. Try to understand how the child feels, what it needs, and assure it that you are now going to be there for it and do everything you can to meet those needs. Imagine you had kept a child in a basement for years and now have to help it believe that you really do care, and that it will never go back in the basement again. This metaphor can help you understand how much work you may have to do to get your Inner Child to trust you.

9. Be sure to conclude the session by reassuring the Inner Child that you love him/her, are always going to be there for them from now on, and are no longer going to deny what they are feeling.

When you first begin doing this exercise you may feel as if you are only acting. That's okay, because there are a million things you can say and there is a reason that you are saying what you are saying. In other words, even if you feel like you are making it up, there is an unconscious reason you are making up specifically what you are. At first you may have trouble getting in touch with your Inner Child, but he/she is always listening. Making this effort will cause them to become more receptive to making contact in future sessions.

As you begin doing these sessions, you may get a sense of distrust from your Inner Child. Again, using the analogy of the child that was kept in the basement for years, trust is not going to be earned overnight but will be earned in time through the consistency of your adult self.

While actively engaged in the *Fat to Fearless*® process, you must follow through on doing this journal every night going forward (or at least as often as you promised your Inner Child that you would). You must follow through on all of the things you promise your Inner Child you will do. If you do not, it's like putting the child back in the basement after promising you wouldn't, which is going to make it twice as hard for him/her to trust you the next time you decide to take her/him out.

It is also very important when speaking from the Inner Child to go with your gut emotional responses without editing them with your conscious mind. You will find that you may start to write something and then may have a tendency to stop because it does not make sense to your conscious mind. Do it anyway, because emotions and feelings in your subconscious are usually not rational, and rationalizing away what you are feeling is one of the ways you have been marginalizing and dishonoring the Inner Child.

This exercise may feel silly, but I assure you that getting in touch with your Inner Child is a very powerful process. Let me give you an example from my own life.

I believe that what you are given to struggle with can turn out to be life's greatest gifts. Overcoming our struggles builds character, creates a deep awakening to self, and often gives us the ability to help others do the same.

For me, the two biggest areas of struggle in my life were my weight and romantic relationships. The problems I have had in both of these areas stemmed back to beliefs of being unlovable, flawed, and not good enough. Changing these core beliefs and overcoming these difficulties led to my life's work and the development of this book, *Fat to Fearless*®, and my book, *Troublesome Attractions*™, written for those who continuously attract unhealthy relationships into their lives.

I was doing this exercise at the end of a relationship with a woman who was completely unsuited for me, was unable to make any type of commitment, and was emotionally abusive at times. Despite my adult, conscious self knowing that she was not a good person to have in my life, I found myself still wanting to be with her. I knew enough to know that this feeling of "want" was coming from my Inner Child.

As a result of these emotions, I ate to self-soothe the loneliness and used food as a substitute for companionship. I quickly gained weight again. I did this exercise to have a better understanding of why my Inner Child still wanted this woman around despite my adult self knowing it wasn't in my best interest. I used my Inner Child Journal to do this. Below is a transcript of my Inner Child journaling session related to this issue:

My Adult: Why do you feel so bad? (Written with my right hand on the right side of the paper; I'm right handed.)

My Inner Child: I'm lonely and I feel like no one really loves me. *(Written with my left hand on the left side of the paper.)*

My Adult: I love you and I want you to know you won't always feel like this.

My Inner Child: It feels like I will. I've always felt like this. I'm never good enough.

My Adult Self: That's because I haven't taken care of you before like I should. I'm so sorry for that and I do love you. I allowed us to become involved with these women that I knew weren't good for us, and because of that you've gotten hurt and come to believe these things that aren't true, that you aren't good enough and are unlovable. You are more than good enough and very lovable and I am going to be here for you and I'm going to help us find someone that doesn't have so many emotional problems and can love us the way we deserve.

My Inner Child: I'm afraid I won't like those people. I won't have the strong feelings I want to have for them like I do her.

My Inner Adult: They won't be the same type of strong feelings because those feelings are based on intensity that you are confusing for love because that's all you've ever known. What you are going to feel for healthy women, for the right woman, is going to feel even better. You may not believe this now, but I'm going to ask you to trust me because I love you and I want what's best for us.

My Inner Child: I just want someone to play with. (This statement came up from within me and when it did, it gave my conscious mind pause. That statement made no sense to me, and I started not to write it, thinking, *That's my conscious mind making that up because it's supposed to be a child and children play, I'm going to disregard that.* But then I caught myself and realized that was exactly what I wasn't supposed to do—let my adult mind come into the process and judge what the Inner Child was saying regardless of how much sense it seemed to make. To do so would have been repressing its thoughts and feelings. That statement had to come from somewhere, so I wrote it down and continued the dialogue.)

My Adult: I don't understand what you mean. You want someone to play with?

My Inner Child: I've never had anyone to play with. No one likes to play with me. I'm afraid these new women will never play with me.

As I continued the dialogue I uncovered that one of the reasons my Inner Child was attracted to these women was that as a child I felt lonely because I had never had any childhood friends. My parents moved frequently for a variety of reasons and we rarely lived anywhere longer than a year, which made forming any significant childhood friendships difficult.

These women all had very wounded Inner Children and underdeveloped adult selves. They were dominated by their Inner Children and were very childlike emotionally. My Inner Child saw them as other children it could befriend. Because they were wounded and damaged too, it believed they wouldn't reject him (my Inner Child).

As you learned with the Symptom Cycle, the way you feel about the problem perpetuates it. My Inner Child's loneliness and low self-esteem was leading me to pick women that I believed would love me but were actually too damaged to ever return that love, thus repeating the cycle.

This Inner Child Journal session provided me with a lot of understanding about why I was attracted to dysfunctional women beyond what I already knew and opened a healing dialogue with my Inner Child that eventually led me to begin attracting healthier partners.

If you are attracted to the wrong people, whether they be abusive or just simply the "wrong ones," be sure to visit my website at www.troublesomeattractions.com for more information on healing and attracting healthy relationships into your life.

The Inner Child Journal is a powerful process to help you get in touch with, understand, and meet the needs of your Inner Child. You will find that allowing it to be heard by communicating with it on a regular basis, many of the negative emotions that you self-soothe through food will subside. Further, when you honor the Inner Child by responding to its needs, you will find that many of these negative emotions are replaced with healthy, life-affirming feelings that support you in your weight loss goals.

SUMMARY

Key Points

- Your Inner Child is your original self. It is who you were when you were born before life experiences caused you to begin to make judgments about how you "should" be.

- Your Inner Child can be thought of as your emotional self.

- Subpersonalities are different "parts" of us that form around different sets of experiences, motivations, and conflicting beliefs. If you've ever argued with yourself, you've had a "parts conflict."

- Most types of parts are always being changed, created, and recreated based on our ongoing experience of living life. However, three parts, often referred to as our primary ego states, tend to stay constant throughout our life unless we take steps to consciously change them at the subconscious level.

- The three primary ego states are the Inner Child, the Inner Critic, and your adult self.

- The one caveat to the above statement about primary ego states changing very little is that the adult self does tend to change in terms of maturity with aging. The Inner Critic and Inner Child, however, remain timelessly the same within the subconscious.

- The Inner Critic develops to ensure you conform with the rules needed to "fit in" to your environment. It typically does this with a negative voice, using the "stick" instead of the "carrot."

- Your Inner Child doesn't go away as you get older; it is typically repressed by the Inner Critic through its constant criticism.

- As you age and become an adult, your adult self tends to lose emotional touch with the Inner Child. Being repressed through the constant criticism of the Inner Critic and forgotten by your adult self leads to the Inner Child having even greater negative emotions that you end up feeling and trying to soothe through food or other unhealthy behaviors.

- To heal the Inner Child you must understand it, which means speaking its language. The Inner Child speaks the language of emotion.

- Whenever you find yourself saying "I want…," "I need…," "It isn't fair…," or "Give me…" in times of strong emotion, it is usually your Inner Child speaking.

- Every time you eat emotionally you are doing so because you are feeling the feelings of the Inner Child within.

- When you don't allow yourself to fully feel your feelings, you are sending the message to your Inner Child that you don't care about its needs. This in turn makes it feel worse. You then feel these negative emotions more strongly the next time, which eventually makes you want to soothe through food or other negative behavior.

- The negative core beliefs you are overcoming are predominantly the beliefs of your Inner Child that you formed in your actual childhood that it has carried over into your adult life.

- To heal your Inner Child and transform its emotions into positive ones you must understand how the three ego states interact. You'll be learning about this in the next chapter.

- One helpful way of thinking about the ego states is that your adult self is your conscious mind while your Inner Critic and Inner Child live in your subconscious.

- The internal subconscious interaction of the Inner Critic and Inner Child are the primary reason for the negative emotions that you try to relieve through food.

- It is the Inner Child that hears and emotionally responds to the criticism of the Inner Critic.

- To stop emotional eating, the Inner Child must be healed of the wounds inflicted from negative childhood events and by the Inner Critic's constant judgment so that it feels good enough to not need food to soothe its emotions.

What This Has To Do With Weight Loss

Learning to communicate with your Inner Child so that you can directly address its emotional needs with something other than food is a skill necessary to stop emotional eating. To truly do this, it helps to learn enough about the Inner Child to allow you to separate from it so that you can identify it, heal it, and eventually reparent and integrate it back into yourself.

You Are Ready To Move To The Next Chapter When . . .

- You have watched the tutorial video for this chapter (if you have the full *Fat to Fearless*® program).

- You have completed the exercises for this chapter in the Success Guide and Workbook (if you have the full *Fat to Fearless*® program).

CHAPTER 19

INTERNAL INTERACTION, EMOTION, AND EATING

Negative emotions do not magically happen; there are things you do within yourself to feel bad, things that happen, that you have never made yourself consciously aware of until now. To feel bad you have to say certain things to yourself and/or make certain pictures in your head. Usually it's a combination of both. This understanding is at the core of Neuro-Linguistic Programming or NLP. NLP—which is often defined as the study of the structure of subjective experience— says that the way we represent things to ourselves, within ourselves, through language, images, internal sounds, and feelings in our body is how we build our emotional states, such as sadness, happiness, fear, and guilt.

Usually you are unconscious of this. You do not realize that every time you feel a specific emotion, you have run the same sequence and done the same things inside of your head that you have done every other time to create that feeling. More often than not, what goes on in those internal dialogues are conversations between the Inner Critic and the Inner Child.

Here is a review of some points about the Inner Critic and the Inner Child.

1. The Inner Child is your original self. It is who you are when you are born. Any time you have childhood trauma, the Inner Child becomes stuck at that age within your subconscious until you do the work to heal that child and fully integrate it into your personality structure.

2. Childhood trauma can be something that, looking back as an adult, might seem benign and harmless. As a child, however, even the simplest events can be misinterpreted and internalized in a way that causes you to form negative opinions and beliefs about yourself and your capabilities. When your adult self looks back on these events, if you can consciously remember them, they may not seem significant; however, your subconscious Inner Child may still be playing out the effects of these events through emotions that you are still feeling today.

3. The Inner Critic developed during early socialization as an inner voice. It is designed to keep you "safe" by keeping you in line with your perceived expectations from your caregivers, peers, and society. Examples include, *Don't show your emotions, fat people aren't liked, be seen and not heard, if you're not perfect, you aren't anything.* These childhood beliefs and expectations are reinforced by the Inner Critic.

4. Since this voice is based on times you were corrected or told to do things differently or be different than you were, the Inner Critic is typically an internalized negative and critical voice based on the worst interpretation of what you perceived your caregivers and peers expected from you as well as your worst interpretation of what they thought of you when you fell short.

Whenever you feel bad about yourself, you are almost always feeling the feelings of the Inner Child. Yet, these feelings do not just automatically happen. They are a direct result of what the Inner Critic says to the Inner Child, which is usually based on some type of external event.

Here is a simple formula for this:

External Stimulus (filtered through negative beliefs and cognitive distortions) + Inner Critic criticizing the Inner Child = negative emotions = emotional self-soothing through food, alcohol, sex, etc.

Let's look at an example:

Shayne has had significant self-esteem and body image issues his entire life. He was raised hearing how good-looking and athletic his brother was, but he was often told that he was not either. He felt bad about himself, and he never did anything to compete with his brother for fear of not measuring up. He feared doing anything athletic because it invited a comparison where he felt he would always come up short.

By avoiding sports and most traditional masculine activities, he only reinforced to himself and others that he was not athletic. The lack of attention from girls that the sports players seem to get just affirmed for him that he was not attractive. By the time Shayne came to see me, he was in his early 20s and about 60 pounds overweight. Over the years, he had gained and lost weight many times, but always fell back into the patterns that led to the overweight body that he now hated himself for having.

When I talked to Shayne, it became very apparent that the primary reason for his overeating was emotional self-soothing as well as an inability to stick with an exercise program for very long. He reported that exercising actually made him more depressed and caused him to eat more.

I understood what was going on with Shayne in the broad sense, but what I needed to know was what was going on inside that caused the emotions that led to him not exercising and overeating. I needed to know what his internal dialogue was.

Below is the transcript of an intake I did with Shayne. I wanted to understand his internal dialogue. Everywhere he indicated he was saying something to himself, hearing a voice in his head, or experiencing a feeling, I made a note to indicate whether it was his Inner Child or his Inner Critic speaking.

Asher: Shayne, today I want to specifically address your issues around exercising. You've told me that you frequently start exercise programs, but within a matter of days to at most weeks you end up quitting, feeling worse than you did when you began, and then usually start binge eating. Is that correct?

Shayne: That's fairly accurate. After I quit the exercise program my eating habits are usually pretty bad, but what I would call binge eating is what I do after my workouts. Of course, I really shouldn't even call them that because usually when I do the binge eating I didn't even finish my workout before I left the gym because I was feeling so bad about myself.

Asher: Let me make sure I understand. You feel motivated to go to the gym, but after you get there you end up feeling really bad about yourself, leave early, and then come home to binge eat. Is that correct?

Shayne: Yes. That doesn't happen every time, but I would say it happens about half the time, which is more than enough for me to not get results, and then overall become discouraged and quit my program.

Asher: Shayne, what exactly is it that happens in between you being motivated enough to go to the gym and then feeling bad about yourself and leaving the gym?

Shayne: I don't know. I guess I just look around at all of the fit and in-shape guys and tell myself that I'm never going to look like that (I know this is the voice of Shayne's Inner Critic).

Asher: So when you get to the gym, you see guys that you perceive are in better shape than you, and then you tell yourself that you're never going to look like that. After you say that to yourself, what happens next?

Shayne: Well, usually I just get this really bad feeling inside. Like I know I don't compare and I'm just not good enough

*and I feel like there's no point (This is his Inner Child emotion-
ally responding to the previous statements he mentioned that
are from his Inner Critic). I usually try to stay for a while by
reminding myself that I know exercise works and if I can just
stick with it I can look like that (this is the voice of his adult self
trying to use reason to motivate him, but as you have learned,
emotion always overpowers reason), but then that other voice
inside just keeps saying that I'll never look like these guys
(Inner Critic), I'm just not masculine enough (Inner Critic),
and I just get this feeling inside like "I know I'm a loser" (the
Inner Child responding to what the Inner Critic just said), and
then I just continue to feel even worse until I leave.*

*Then usually as soon as I get home, the first thing I do is
eat something like ice cream and watch TV to try to feel better
(the Inner Child feels bad now and wants to feel better). Of
course that only works for a little while because after I'm done
binge eating, I start telling myself what a complete failure I
am (Inner Critic and also the Symptom Cycle at work), which
just makes me feel even worse and I end up drinking or going
to bed early or even eating more (continued Inner Child emotional response).*

From this interaction, you can see the structure of how your
Inner Child and Inner Critic interact to produce bad feelings.
You can also see the Symptom Cycle at work again in that his
bad feelings about himself creates emotions that when acted on
perpetuate the reason he feels bad to begin with.

Your Inner Critic, the voice that reinforces your negative
and limiting core beliefs, responds to anything in the environment that triggers an opportunity to reinforce those beliefs.
Your Inner Child responds by feeling bad, and when those
emotions grow strong enough, your Inner Child overwhelms
your reasoning adult self with emotion and takes over. Once in
control of your behavior, your Inner Child wants to do something to feel better in the quickest way possible. For those who
struggle with weight, food is usually the quickest fix.

Let's look at another example:

Bridget was a 28-year-old corporate real estate agent that had a weight problem. Part of her job required her to frequently attend after-hours functions with prospective clients. She would plan in advance when she had to go out to one of these events and what her healthy meal choices would be. She also committed herself to having no alcoholic beverages. However, that almost never happened.

Bridget had been raised in an environment where she came to believe that to be liked you had to be fun, and if she was not fun, no one would like her. This negative core belief, that people liking her was based on how exciting and entertaining she was as opposed to who she really was as a person, was reinforced by the Inner Critic.

These events frequently began with her sticking to her healthy decisions, but every time there was a lull in the conversation where she sensed any type of disapproval from others, her Inner Critic would tell her things like, You're no fun when you don't drink. If you drink, they will like you more. They think you're no fun because you're not eating dessert with them.

This caused her Inner Child to panic, since one of its childhood wounds was the negative core belief that she would not be liked if she was not fun, and fun was about participating (this was also combined with some childhood abandonment fears). These fears and emotions from her Inner Child, coupled with the reinforcing negative criticism of the Inner Critic, would overwhelm her adult decision-making abilities. She would find herself indulging in the very thing she had promised herself she would not: food and high-calorie alcohol.

As you know from the Symptom Cycle, the things you do to soothe the negative emotions only reinforce the negative core beliefs and lead to more negative emotions that result in more negative behaviors. Every time this happened, she would lose confidence in herself, gain more weight, and feel more hopeless and out of control.

How do you change this internal dialogue so that it doesn't lead to the emotions that cause you to turn to food to feel better? Stopping this downward spiral of negative emotions and self-soothing behavior is a two-step process:

1. Disempower the Inner Critic so that it has less impact on the Inner Child. You are already actively doing this by:

   • Confronting the critic and its cognitive distortions and uncovering the truth behind its lies.

   • Using submodality changes to alter the audio qualities of the voice while also assigning it a humorous caricature so that it's difficult to take what it says seriously.

   • Actively working to change the negative core beliefs that motivate its criticism.

2. Reparent the Inner Child and provide it with what it needs emotionally. Allow it to feel good about itself in a way that does not cause it to need to act out with self-soothing and self-destructive behaviors.

You are already making the Inner Child feel better by giving it new, healthier beliefs as well as beginning to communicate with it through your Inner Child Journal. Next you will learn how to reparent your Inner Child and help heal the emotions that resulted from its old limiting core beliefs and the negative perception of childhood events that helped form them.

EXERCISE: EMOTIONAL MOMENTS REVIEW

In this exercise you are going to track any periods of feeling negative emotions over the next week and begin to see how they correspond to interactions between your Inner Critic and Inner Child.

Do this exercise in your Success Guide and Workbook.

1. Throughout the week, any time you feel bad, especially if these feelings make you want to turn to food, immediately stop what you're doing and become fully present in the moment.

2. Review what was going on in your mind before you started feeling bad. Specifically, what were your thoughts? Based on what you've learned, can you attribute these thoughts to the Inner Critic?

3. Once you've identified what the Inner Critic said, log the emotions that followed. Can you get a sense of the almost childlike hurt behind these feelings?

4. If possible, immediately use your Inner Child Journal to dialogue with your Inner Child about these feelings. When your adult self responds to your Inner Child, be sure to:

   • Assure the Inner Child that it is loved and whatever it concluded from what the Inner Critic said is not true. Through your affirmations, provide your Inner Child with the truth about its value and worth.

   • Ask the Inner Child what you can do to make it feel better. If it responds with food, ask it what else you can give it that would make it feel better instead. It's important to explain to the Inner Child that the reason you do not want to give it food is that you know in the long run food will just make him/her feel worse and you love your Inner Child too much for that.

5. Continue to do this past this week and it will eventually become habit. This is a healthy way for you to soothe the Inner Child other than with food. Also, if you make an agreement with yourself to do this every time before you eat emotionally you will soon find by the time the exercise is over the urge has passed.

SUMMARY

Key Points

- Almost every time you feel bad about yourself it is the result of your Inner Child personalizing the criticism of the Inner Critic. Your adult self has more intellectual defenses built up against this criticism, but your Inner Child doesn't have any more defense mechanisms to protect itself now than you did when you were an actual child.

- Put simply, your strong and chronic negative emotions emanate from the Inner Child as a result of feeling criticized and attacked by the Inner Critic.

- Eventually, the Inner Child feels bad enough that it overwhelms your reasoning mind with emotion and takes control of your behavior. In an attempt to alleviate the pain, it does whatever it can to feel better as quickly as possible. For most with weight issues, food is usually the first choice.

- This self-soothing behavior only leaves you feeling worse and reinforces your negative core beliefs. It fuels the cycle to happen over and over again.

- An equation to help you understand how this interaction between the Inner Critic and the Inner Child leads to emotional eating is:

  External Stimulus (filtered through negative beliefs and cognitive distortions) + Inner Critic criticizing the Inner Child = negative emotions = emotional self-soothing through food, alcohol, sex, etc.

- When looking at the interaction between the Inner Critic and the Inner Child you can also see the Symptom Cycle playing out. Remember the Symptom Cycle says that the way we feel about the symptom (being overweight) creates feelings that when acted upon (emotional eating) creates and reinforces the original reason for the bad feelings (being overweight) while constantly recycling and reinforcing your negative core beliefs.

What This Has To Do With Weight Loss

When you make subconscious processes conscious, you gain the ability to influence and change them. By learning to become aware of the internal dialogue between the Inner Critic and Inner Child and the emotions that result from this dialogue, you begin to gain control over your own emotions, including the ones that in the past have motivated you to eat for reasons other than hunger and good nutrition.

You Are Ready To Move To The Next Chapter When . . .

- You can begin to observe this internal dialogue within yourself and see the emotional impact it has. Ideally, you can identify this dialogue specifically in moments where you're tempted to eat emotionally. Using this chapter's exercise with what you've already learned can begin soothing your child in ways other than with food.

- You have watched the tutorial video for this chapter (if you have the full *Fat to Fearless*® program).

- You have completed the exercises for this chapter in the Success Guide and Workbook (if you have the full *Fat to Fearless*® program).

CHAPTER 20

REPARENTING THE INNER CHILD

The term "reparenting" in traditional psychological circles refers to a series of techniques devised in the late 1960s by social worker, Jacqui Schiff. In this version, the client would relive their childhood with their therapist acting as a stand-in for their parent. The therapist acted as a healthy parent in these relived situations. The therapist's job was to provide what the client did not receive in their actual childhood, and in theory this would help heal their emotional wounds. This type of reparenting, however, has fallen into disrepute and is generally deemed as ineffective.

One of the reasons this type of reparenting had limited success was that the "healthy parent" was only available during the actual sessions with the client. However, the client's Inner Critic was always with them, providing an emotionally abusive and pessimistic soundtrack to life 24 hours a day.

The type of reparenting you will do is very different from this because your adult self is going to take over the role of parenting your Inner Child. Much like the Inner Critic, your adult self is there all the time to safeguard the Inner Child's best interests. To reparent your Inner Child, your adult conscious self meets the Inner Child's emotional needs that were not met in childhood in a way that allows the Inner Child to heal while feeling loved and cared for by your adult self.

One of the most difficult parts of this process is that for most of us who have denied their Inner Child's needs for most of our adult lives, our Inner Child is not very trusting of our adult selves. Being overweight for any extended period of time is proof that you have neglected your Inner Child. Otherwise, it would not have needed to eat to feel better.

As a healthy adult parenting a child in a healthy way, you would have been in touch with your child's emotional needs enough to soothe them while also setting healthy boundaries around food. If you are the actual parent of an actual overweight child, these same lessons can be applied to your children to help them feel valued and not turn to food to feel good.

Earning your Inner Child's trust will be key to your success in reparenting, as will consistency in the way you treat your Inner Child and intervene to protect it from the Inner Critic.

The most important aspect of reparenting your Inner Child is communicating with it on a regular basis, and going within daily to make sure that it feels heard, loved, valued and taken care of. A great way of understanding this is to think about the last time you really felt bad emotionally. This may have been a time that you had this sinking feeling in your chest or a hurt in the pit of your stomach. Those emotional responses are your Inner Child. Often the Inner Child communicates through feelings in the body.

You may remember wishing you could feel better, that you could somehow get in touch with that feeling and change it. The feeling of being disconnected from your ability to understand and change how you feel in a hurtful situation is an example of being disconnected from your Inner Child (essentially being disconnected from your emotional self). Once you have done the work of reparenting and have a relationship with your Inner Child, you will never be out of touch with your feelings again or unable to have an impact on your emotional state unless you go back to your previous behavior of ignoring and repressing the Inner Child's needs and emotions.

You have dishonored your Inner Child any time you have not completely acknowledged and owned all of your feelings. Usually, this is because those feelings are being repressed by the Inner Critic, which is making your adult mind believe that the criticism is valid and deserved. To be whole, to be complete, you must honor all of yourself and feel all of your feelings completely without judgment.

Whenever you judge a part of yourself as bad or unacceptable and then deny it, you give it power over you. It is like a beach ball held underwater. The deeper you take it, the more force it exerts trying to rise to the surface. The longer you keep it underwater, the more tired you become holding it down. Eventually it breaks free.

Emotions work the same way. Whenever you try to suppress or keep from feeling a part of yourself, you become tired from the effort, and at some point that emotion surfaces, often in unexpected ways and at less than ideal times. Also, because the emotion has been suppressed, just like the ball forcefully pops out of the water, these emotions often erupt to the surface with an intensity inappropriate to the actual situation that triggered them.

Being emotionally whole and complete is also at the heart of good decision-making and healthy intuition. It allows you to be in touch with all of your needs and all of the internal resources you were born to have. It allows you to make decisions motivated by what is in your best interest, not decisions based on avoiding dealing with parts of yourself that you've denied. Being in touch with all of your emotions, honoring and feeling them fully, is also at the heart of healing your Inner Child and the chronic negative emotions it feels when it is neglected and denied. The emotions that often cause you to reach for unhealthy foods.

When you were a child, the same experiences that led to the formation of your negative core beliefs, also had you believing that part of you was unacceptable. You might have learned that expressing anger made you unlovable, or that if you had too many needs it was too much of a burden for those around you. You learned to suppress those needs and the feelings that went with them.

Part of the development of those negative core beliefs was also the development of the Inner Critic, which acted as your internal taskmaster to ensure your behavior kept you in line with those beliefs. This included ensuring you did not feel any emotions that were deemed wrong. Since these were the emotions of the Inner Child, you learned to believe that part of you was unacceptable. Every time the Inner Critic causes you to deny your feelings, you are denying and disowning the Inner Child part of yourself.

Have you ever been in a situation where you wanted to cry, be angry, or stand up for yourself? You wanted to express that you were hurt, but you did not do it because the voice of the Inner Critic told you that you shouldn't? Maybe it sounded something like, *Don't be a baby, suck it up and show them how strong you are, don't let anyone see that you're hurt, they will think less of you,* or *don't say what you're really feeling or they'll think you're needy and they might leave you."*

Every time you have done this, you have been denying part of yourself. You have been ignoring the Inner Child and making it feel worse by telling it that its needs are not important. That she/he is wrong for feeling what it does. When you've done this, you've caused your Inner Child to strongly feel the negative emotions of sadness, hurt, neglect, and anxiety that led you to reach for food to soothe its pain.

Put simply, you may believe that the feelings of rejection and believing you're not good enough are based on how you perceive the world and how those around you feel about you, but that's actually a projection. The truth is that those are feelings your Inner Child is experiencing based on how it perceives you feel about him or her.

It is helpful to think of your Inner Child as if it were a real child. Imagine if every time your child had any feelings you did not think they should have, you either ignored them and made no attempts to make them feel better or told them they were "wrong" for having the feelings. What type of impact do you think that would have on their self-esteem? They would learn that they were unimportant, not good enough, that their needs did not matter and they couldn't trust their own instincts and intuition about their own feelings or themselves.

That is what your Inner Child learned when you did not honor all of your feelings. This disowned Inner Child is the source of your own low self-esteem. Integral to the process of healing your Inner Child is to honor it by allowing it to have all of its emotions and still accept and love them fully.

You might think that some emotions are bad. Why would you want to feel anger, for instance? The belief that any part of you is bad is an idea that you got from childhood. It is at the root of many people's chronic issues. When you believe that you are flawed in some intrinsic way, that is the childhood belief that you have been soothing your entire life.

Emotions by themselves are not bad. Sometimes the behaviors that result from certain emotions are less than ideal, but that too is a result of not balancing those emotions with a loving and nurturing adult self. Even those less-than-ideal behaviors can lead to circumstances that promote self-growth and healing if you keep your eyes open and try to become more conscious through the process.

Anger is the emotion that most of my clients suppress the most. They learned in childhood to suppress their own needs and put others before themselves. They believed this would make them lovable and bring them the acknowledgment and appreciation they so desperately wanted.

The only way to chronically put others' needs before your own is to avoid feeling the resentment and anger that eventually builds up inside. It is a no-win situation. To feel truly happy you have to feel loved, accepted, and appreciated. If you believe the only way for that to happen is for you to put others before you and deny your own wants and needs, this will lead to anger and resentment that you deny and suppress.

This then leads to low self-esteem, depression, and self-soothing behavior—including food, drugs, sex, and spending—that makes you even more unhappy and reinforces your lack of self-worth.

However, anger can be a positive emotion that leads to positive assertiveness when guided by your healthy adult self. It can help you stand up for your rights and what you deserve in a way that honors all of you while not dishonoring anyone else.

It is impossible to have healthy self-esteem without having assertiveness and it is impossible to be assertive if you do not feel your anger. Our emotions are like guidance systems for a happy life. What you feel tells you if you are headed in the right direction toward fulfillment. Without feeling anger, you would never know that you were being wronged or dishonoring yourself.

Extreme anger can be destructive, but usually it is a result of many instances that have built over time where you have not attended to your own interests, wants, and needs. Often, you are also subconsciously feeling anger toward yourself for not looking out for yourself first.

When you use anger as the spark for healthy assertiveness, you send a message to your subconscious that you deserve to be treated well. When you do this, anger rarely has a chance to build to the point of being destructive.

This is true for all of your emotions, not just anger. Sadness, guilt, and fear all have a healthy role in helping you build the life you want. These emotions only become a problem when you either give them power over yourself by suppressing them, or when you go to the other extreme and habitually wallow in them so that you see all of life through a very limited set of emotions. You can't be happy being anything less than yourself, and you can't fully be yourself without feeling the full spectrum of all of your feelings.

In the next set of exercises in your *Fat to Fearless*® journey, you will learn to give yourself permission to feel all of your emotions as well as begin reparenting your Inner Child.

EXERCISE: INNER CHILD HYPNOTHERAPY

One of the most powerful ways of reparenting your Inner Child is to use your *Fat to Fearless*® Inner Child Hypnotherapy Audio Session.

In this session you will explore all of your feelings and feel them fully and completely. This can be a powerfully emotional process, and it is recommended that when you first do this session that you have plenty of time and do not have to go anywhere afterward for at least one hour. When the session is over, give yourself the opportunity to sit with your feelings and allow for emotional integration.

In this session you will go into hypnosis and meet your Inner Child. You will ask key questions that will give you information as to what your Inner Child needs to feel loved and why it drives you to overeat. As you ask and receive answers, it will feel heard and loved.

This session will also provide positive reinforcement for your Inner Child, acknowledging its value and allowing it to feel loved and heard. You may find yourself returning to this session many times over, at first because of the Inner Child's need to heal, and then afterwards because of how good it feels to acknowledge and love all of your emotional self.

Follow the instructions that accompany this audio session and you will find yourself on your way to healing your Inner Child.

EXERCISE: EMOTIONAL LIBERATION

One of the reasons your Inner Child feels wounded and unheard is because your Inner Critic has repressed many of its emotions through constant criticism. Eventually, it just gave up on allowing itself to experience these feelings after a lifetime of emotional neglect and being told it was "wrong" to have them.

Liberating these emotions and learning to feel all of them fully and completely is necessary for the Inner Child, and for you to feel whole and complete. One way for you to determine how much these emotions have been repressed is to understand the concept of resonance.

Sounds in music resonate and intensify in the presence of a sympathetic vibration. Events and emotions resonate when they strike a chord with what you already believe or with feelings you already have. When you have repressed emotion, just like the beach ball being held underwater, they are very near the surface and ready to "pop up" at the first opportunity. When you are exposed to things that are sympathetic (similar) to the emotions that you are repressing, the amplification of those inner emotions is felt very strongly. Let's look at some practical examples:

Have you ever watched a movie, television show, or even a commercial and felt overwhelmed by strong emotion that seemed out of proportion to what you were watching?

Have you ever listened to a story and felt overwhelmed by feelings that seemed out of proportion to what was being expressed in the narrative?

Do you feel strong emotions that you feel disconnected from, and you do not understand why you are feeling them to the degree that you are?

If the answer is yes to any of the above questions, then these experiences are resonating with your repressed emotions that you are disconnected from but are just below the surface. Learning to express these emotions is key to your healing, but it is also important to get out all of those emotions you have already stored in your body.

Negative emotions such as anger or guilt that are repressed long enough and not vented, eventually lead to all types of illnesses, including cancer. It is time to purge these repressed emotions, and then allow your ongoing emotions to flow freely. This is sometimes referred to as cathartic emotional release. I call this process Emotional Liberation.

While releasing your repressed emotions can certainly be cathartic, all cathartic emotional release work is not about liberating repressed emotions. Some cathartic emotional release work can be about not wanting to feel negative or uncomfortable emotions, which just perpetuates the problem.

For example, when you are angry and take a baseball bat and beat your bed, this would be defined as a cathartic emotional release. However, in this instance the person is trying to get the anger "out" by venting it through their body as opposed to feeling it and processing it. By trying to avoid feeling anger, this type of cathartic emotional release is actually an ineffective form of emotional repression.

In 1990, at Iowa State University, psychologist Brad Bushman began studying emotional release as it pertained to anger. Bushman ran a study with 180 students divided into two groups. Each group was given an essay to write. No matter how good the essay was, they were all given a bad grade.

They were then told that they were going to compete in a contest against the person who graded their essay. The winner of the contest would have the ability to blast their opponent with a loud noise, the volume of which they would get to control.

The first group, after receiving their bad grade and while waiting for the contest to begin, was told to take their anger out on a punching bag. The other group was told to sit, process, and fully feel their anger. What happened?

The group that punched the punching bag turned the volume up 3 times higher when blasting their opponent than the group that sat and felt their anger. Expressing their anger physically as opposed to simply emotionally processing it actually increased their aggressive feelings. In the reverse, those who allowed themselves the opportunity to feel their anger without channeling it outside of themselves had much less remaining animosity toward their opponents by the time the game began. This is why if you choose to do physical work to release emotion that you pair it with time to cognitively and emotionally process it as well.

For this reason, I avoid the term cathartic emotional release, and instead use the term Emotional Liberation. You are not trying to not feel emotions by getting them out, but instead you are liberating the emotions you have stored and trapped within yourself, in many cases for several years.

Below is the process for Emotional Liberation. Only a few emotions have been listed here, but this process can be used for any emotion you are not fully allowing yourself to feel.

1. Make a list of as many emotions as you can think of, especially the ones that you seem to feel the least often.

2. For each emotion, write down experiences in your life when you have felt that emotion, even if only a small amount, as well as times that you didn't feel these emotions in situations that your objective mind believes it would have been appropriate.

3. Make plans to engage in activities, one whole week of activities per emotion, designed to bring that emotion up and express it fully and completely.

4. Be sure to actively journal through the process, paying particular attention to the Inner Critic's judgments about these emotions or the process. Disempower the Inner Critic through the techniques you have already learned and add to your conscious awareness the ways that you have observed the Inner Critic trying to repress these emotions.

Below are some examples as well as a deeper understanding of the importance of resolving guilt.

Liberate Sadness. Rent every sad movie you can get your hands on, the worst tearjerkers ever made, and spend a whole week watching as many of them as you can. Cry as much as possible and really let the tears flow. If this resonates with sad experiences from your own life, allow yourself to feel that sadness and journal about it. Own your sadness and you will find that it loses its power over you and simply becomes a healthy part of your full emotional palette. I promise you will feel better by the end of the week.

Use your Inner Child Journal nightly to dialogue with your Inner Child about these emotions when they come up. Make sure your Inner Child knows it's okay to feel these feelings and it's part of being emotionally healthy. Be sure to end your journaling by assuring your Inner Child that it's loved and how your new core beliefs (being loveable, worthwhile, etc.) are true.

Liberate Anger. Liberate the anger you are not feeling fully. Make a list of all the times you perceived yourself as having been wronged or trampled upon, with a special emphasis on the ones you feel you should have been more angry about or expressed anger more openly than you did in the situation. Take a picture of the person involved or some symbol that represents the situation and allow yourself to yell, scream, and say all the things you want to or feel you should have said to this person.

Typically this will follow a curve. You may not feel the anger when you start, but if you "fake it 'til you make it," the anger will eventually surface. As you get it all out, it will then subside. You can also use a bat on your bed or other unbreakable things to fully release it from your body. Unlike in the example of using the bat for cathartic emotional release, you are not trying to get out emotions you do not want to feel. You are using the physical movement to bring up and then release emotions stored inside that you are having trouble feeling and have not allowed yourself to express. Do this for a week and you will feel better, lighter, and more full of energy.

Once you've liberated this anger, you can then refer back to the section on forgiveness to release any negativity you may still hold for those involved. You cannot release the anger and use it productively to build healthy assertiveness if you maintain unforgiveness and a victim's mindset.

Use your Inner Child Journal nightly to dialogue with your Inner Child about these emotions when they come up. Make sure your Inner Child knows it's okay to feel these feelings and it's part of being emotionally healthy. Be sure to end your journaling by assuring your Inner Child that it's loved and how your new core beliefs (being loveable, worthwhile, etc.) are true.

Liberate Guilt. Guilt often comes from feeling emotions you think are wrong. Judging our emotions is at the heart of repression and guilt often presides over the process. Releasing this judgment, this guilt, is necessary because it is often the cap on top of all the other emotions you repress. For example, if you think only bad people get angry, your guilt about expressing anger is one of the mechanisms that represses that anger. Likewise, if you have negative feelings toward people that you believe you should never feel badly about, like your parents, you experience guilt that keeps you from expressing the emotions you need to feel and release, which just intensifies these emotions and the guilt that comes with them.

Step 1

Make a list of every event in your life that has caused you to feel anger that you judge as inappropriate. Put each one on a separate sheet of paper and write a brief reason why you feel you should feel guilty about this event.

Step 2

Search this narrative for cognitive distortions and see how this changes the story.

For example, perhaps your parents did something to you that causes you to feel anger toward them. You judge yourself as "wrong" for feeling that anger because no one should ever feel anger or hatred toward their parents. When you go through this you realize that "no one should ever" is a cognitive distortion in that it is an over generalization. When you think about it you realize that there are certainly circumstances where people should feel anger toward their parents, and whether deserved or not—you do feel anger—and until you acknowledge this and allow yourself to feel the anger, you always will.

You will frequently have emotions toward a person that you feel is inappropriate for this particular person. Often, this takes the form of anger or hate toward a parent. If you feel you have been wronged, anger is a natural human response. You should not judge yourself for having that response. By judging it, you are repressing it. To heal something, you must feel it. To no longer have anger or hatred for someone, you must reach forgiveness. But you can never forgive if you do not first experience and then move through anger. The key is to not get stuck in it. By realizing that feeling the full spectrum of human emotions is part of the human experience, you give yourself permission to own your feelings. You forgive yourself for judging your emotions and releasing the guilt. When you do this you will typically find that not only the guilt disappears, but because you allowed yourself to feel that anger without judgment, the anger has dissipated as well. Often, after allowing yourself to feel and release the anger, you are also able to see the situation more clearly, which not only leads to forgiveness but also peace.

Step 3
Make a list of things that you have done that you feel guilty about and ask yourself the following questions:

a. Can I separate myself from my behavior? Can I see that what I did, while maybe not a choice I would make now, does not define me or determine who I am as a person?

b. Was I evil or just doing the best I could in the situation?

c. Have there been situations in my life where I have been wronged and I have forgiven others?

d. Knowing that I was just doing the best I could, and would make a different choice now, can I choose to extend the forgiveness to myself that I have extended others?

If the answers to these questions allow you to forgive yourself, ritualistically tear up or burn the paper you've written these events down on as a symbol of resolution. If possible and appropriate, ask for forgiveness from those you have wronged. You can also write a letter (one you never send) to the person who was wronged if actual contact is not possible. This allows for an internal dialogue of forgiveness that can provide much relief from guilt. Once you've released these emotions, you not only find that you feel better emotionally but physically as well, as your body does not have to carry all of those repressed feelings.

EXERCISE: NLP REPARENTING

The NLP Neurological Reparenting Process has proven to be very effective to help rewire neurology related to unmet childhood needs and the emotions those needs produce today through your unhealed Inner Child. It takes advantage of your brain's inability to distinguish between real and imagined experiences if the imagined experiences have enough emotion attached to them.

With this technique you can change your painful childhood experiences by combining them with the strengths and experiences you have had as an adult. This is a very powerful technique and I recommend practicing it as often as possible. Also, be sure to watch the instructional video for this exercise.

Step 1

List your top three limiting beliefs you want to change and the positive core beliefs you want to replace them with.

Examples:

I'm not good enough *becomes* I'm more than good enough.

I'm unlovable *becomes* I am lovable.

The harder I try, the more I fail *becomes* I am always rewarded for my effort.

Step 2

For each of your negative core beliefs, think of your earliest memory or experience where you remember feeling that belief. For example, if one of your negative core beliefs is *not being good enough*, your earliest conscious memory of that may be an instance in childhood where a parent criticized you while simultaneously praising a sibling. It is not necessary to write down these memories in detail, just write down enough to remind you of the memory you are going to use for that specific core belief.

Ideally, all of these memories will be from childhood, as this core belief was most likely formed then. The earlier the memories, the greater the impact this technique has. If you can only remember more recent experiences, go ahead and use those. Often we block out troubled periods of our life and many of my clients only have hazy recollections of their childhood when we begin working together. As you continue to do this work and bring up more unconscious material, new memories will most likely surface and this technique can then be applied to those memories. Examples of possible negative core beliefs and the associated memories are below.

Examples:

> I am not good enough.
> *Dad criticized me at the park and praised my sister.*

> I am unlovable.
> *I was sad about skinning my knee, and Mom wouldn't hold me and told me to "toughen up."*

> The harder I try, the more I fail.
> *I worked all night on my science project, and Dad told me it was stupid.*

Step 3

For each of the positive core beliefs you want to install instead of the negative core beliefs above, think of the strongest memory you have of having felt this way.

Examples:

> I am more than good enough.
> *My first boyfriend chose me over all my friends to ask to the dance.*

> I am lovable.
> *My sister's speech at my wedding about how much she loves me.*

> I am always rewarded for my effort.
> *I was promoted and they wrote an article about me in the newsletter.*

Step 4

Now you are going to create an anchor, and then stack these positive feelings of the beliefs you want to have onto this anchor. This allows you to take these positive feelings back into your old memories and change the way your brain processes them.

Anchoring is an NLP technique that associates emotional states with gestures, touches, or sounds that enable these emotional states to be recalled at will by consciously doing the gesture, applying the touch, or hearing the sound. It is very much like Pavlov and his dogs. By ringing the bell every time he gave them food and they salivated, he was eventually able to ring the bell and they would salivate without even giving them the food. The bell became their anchor for salivating.

You can also think of anchors from your own experience. Have you ever been driving and a song came on the radio that gave you an immediate emotional reaction? Maybe it took you back to a place and time where you first heard the song and associated positive feelings with it? This is an example of an anchor. Every time you are exposed to the stimulus (the song) it produces a response (the feelings and/or memory recall). But what would happen if you heard this song and it triggered the positive emotions *while you were doing something that you currently associate with negative feelings?*

If this happened often enough, your brain would begin to become confused about this experience that you currently label as "negative" because—with the help of the song—you would be feeling positive feelings while doing it. In this confusion, you actually have the choice, if you know how, of being able to change and re-code the previously developed neurological association your brain made between the current experience and the negative feelings. Using this same principle, we can "confuse" your brain into re-coding past traumatic events to be at the very least more neutral, while layering positive experiences on top of them.

To begin, you want an anchor you can use to recall at any time the positive beliefs you chose above and the feelings you associate with them. First, we want to choose a kinesthetic (touch) anchor that you can apply anytime you want. It can be anything, but it should be something you do not do regularly or it will desensitize the anchor if done too often. For your first anchor, you will touch your right thumb and forefinger together. (If you are left-handed, use your left thumb and forefinger). If for some reason you already do the suggested anchors frequently, just create one of your own. The video tutorial will explain this in detail.

Step 5

A. Recall the first positive memory. Make sure you are associated in the memory, which means seeing it through your own eyes. Use all of your senses to make this memory as real as possible until you are actually feeling them as if you were there. When you feel it is at its strongest point and you are fully feeling the emotions you associate with this positive memory, set your anchor. When you set an anchor, you perform the kinesthetic touch at the peak of the emotional experience you want to pair with the anchor. Hold your anchor for five seconds, and then release it.

With the anchor we've chosen, you will, at the peak of the positive feelings, touch your right thumb and forefinger together for five seconds while saying to yourself (or out loud) the positive belief you've associated with this memory. It also helps to take deep breaths during this process, as the breathing becomes another anchor within itself to this positive state (don't, however, use the breathing to anchor the negative state when you get to that step below).

B. Now you want to break the state. This means do something to return to a more neutral way of feeling. Maybe flip through a magazine, try to recall what you had for breakfast last Tuesday, or mentally review your schedule for tomorrow. Spend no more than 30 seconds doing this.

C. Now repeat step A and B two more times. By the time you are done, you will have associated into the memory and set your anchor three times, breaking the state in between.

D. Now let's test your anchor. Going from a neutral state, fire your anchor. Firing an anchor is when you perform the gesture to intentionally create the response within you that you anchored. For our purposes, without consciously recalling the memory associated to the good feeling and positive belief, touch your thumb and forefinger together and say your positive core belief and notice how the positive feeling returns without having to consciously recall the memory. You have now anchored that positive feeling and new belief to the action of touching your thumb and forefinger together.

E. Now repeat the above instructions A through E for the other two positive memories using the same anchor as the first positive memory (thumb and forefinger). This is called stacking anchors, which means that you are stacking emotions (or technically any state of response) on top of others on the same anchor so that when the anchor is fired, it will trigger all of the positive states and emotions at the same time.

Step 6

Now, after testing your positive anchor to make sure it works, break your state so that you are more emotionally neutral and go back into the first negative memory you associated with a core belief you want to change. You will now anchor the negative feelings using the forefinger and thumb of your other hand. (If you are right-handed, it will be your left forefinger and thumb that you use.) In the example used above, you would go back to the memory of your dad criticizing you and praising your sister and anchor with your left hand the feeling of not being good enough.

Test the negative anchor before moving on. You should be able to recall the negative feelings just by firing the anchor without actually recalling the memory.

Unlike the positive anchors, where we stacked all of the good feelings and beliefs on top of each other, you will only anchor the feelings and beliefs from one of the negative memories before moving to the next step.

Step 7

You have now anchored all three positive emotional responses and beliefs on your right hand and the first negative belief and related emotions on your left hand. Now close your eyes and go back to that first negative memory and fire the anchor for the negative emotion and belief. This should bring forth the feeling of not being good enough, etc.

Now, while still holding the negative anchor, fire the positive stacked-anchor on your other hand, breathe deeply, and let those positive emotions overwhelm the negative ones. At this point you are holding both anchors.

*If you took deep breaths while creating your positive anchor, begin doing so now as well.

Step 8

Release the negative anchor first, and while still holding the positive anchor, allow your adult conscious mind to come into the scene and tell this younger you what he or she needs to hear to affirm to your Inner Child that the new positive core belief is true. In our example, your adult conscious mind would tell the younger you in this memory that he or she is more than good enough. Hugging the child in your mind is also helpful, as the feeling of love and human touch amplifies all of the other positive emotions.

Another variation of this exercise is to simply reimagine the scene as you wish it had been. Simply change the events, rewriting history, so that your Inner Child feels loved, supported, etc. from your reimagined version. This technique also takes advantage of the subconscious' inability to separate real events from ones imagined with enough emotion.

Once you have done this in one of the two ways described above, release the positive anchor at the peak of the positive emotion. This may be at the point at which you are hugging the younger you.

Step 9

Give yourself five to ten minutes to assimilate this experience. You have now started to change some of your earliest neurological imprints by mixing them with later positive experiences. You are breaking up the neurological structure of events that lead to beliefs that lead to emotions that have, as a neurological bundle, helped to maintain these negative core beliefs.

While you sit and allow yourself to process this experience, it can be helpful to recall all the other times in your life that you felt the positive emotion and belief. This would also be a great time to review your evidence journal. I also like to spend the last minute of this reflection time repeating my affirmations to myself.

Step 10

Repeat these steps for the other two negative memories and try to practice this technique at least once a day for four weeks. Each week you can switch to a different set of negative memories that you want to change.

In John Bradshaw's book *Homecoming*, he elaborates on this technique by having you choose different negative memories from each psychosocial stage of development. *Homecoming* is a book entirely about reparenting the Inner Child and is an excellent resource for those who want more insight into this technique beyond the scope of what the *Fat to Fearless®* program currently offers without private sessions with myself or one of my online coaching programs. Also, to better understand all of the steps, be sure to watch the video demonstration included in the full *Fat to Fearless®* program of me performing NLP reparenting with an actual client.

EXERCISE: INNER CHILD DAY

A great way to honor your Inner Child is to celebrate it with an Inner Child Day. An Inner Child Day is a day that you spend exclusively doing activities that your Inner Child wants to do. Your role as a healthy adult is simply to joyously participate without judging the activities as childish. Below are some great examples of things you can do on your Inner Child Day:

1. Go to an amusement park, but keep it stress-free and fun.

2. Play video games.

3. Put together puzzles or play board games with other friends that are having their Inner Child day as well.

4. Give your child special treats that it's been saving to have on Inner Child Day.

5. Buy yourself toys from your childhood. (I once bought Transformer toys from the '80s on eBay but waited for my Inner Child Day to open them.)

6. Go to the park and swing and slide and other fun child-like activities.

The list of things you may want to do are personal to your own Inner Child. The key is to enjoy them without judging them or feeling any negative emotions at all. For example, do not feel guilt for spending the day on something that your adult self might judge as foolish or a waste of time.

Decide how often it is best for you to have an Inner Child Day. I recommend once a month, but have one at the very least every three months. If giving your child permission to eat outside of your healthy eating plan is part of your Inner Child Day as opposed to just simply one or two treats, then it may be best to do it every three months to avoid a relapse of using food to self-soothe. This will help you keep it as a happy reward to celebrate how wonderful and loved your child is.

Below is a photo that I took on my first Inner Child Day, which I celebrated with a close friend's Inner Child as well. Whenever possible, it is always best to share an Inner Child day with others, since playing with others and healthy socialization is at the heart of being a child. Both of us had been craving a "big cookie" from the mall for months, and we decided that was what we would get our Inner Children as a treat for the day. The icing on the cookie reads "Happy Inner Child Day From Subie." (Subie was the nickname for our subconscious minds.)

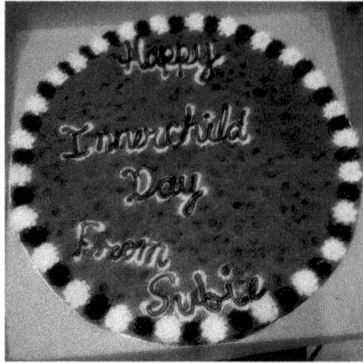

If you have children of your own, letting your Inner Child play with them for a day is a wonderful way of deepening your connection with your children while also giving your Inner Child someone to play with. Find your own unique ways to celebrate your Inner Child and make your own Inner Child Day special.

Strengthening Your Adult Self

Of your three primary ego states, the one that I have talked the least about is your adult self. Your adult self is the rational, logical, and planning part of yourself. Typically, your adult self is an unwitting hostage to the interactions between your Inner Child and Inner Critic, yet it is important to state that your "adult" has a job to do as well and often needs strengthening to do that job.

Your adult self is usually the "you" of which you are conscious. While it is very much the thinking part of you, it is not devoid of emotion.

Your adult self certainly feels, yet those emotions are less rooted in the past, such as with the Inner Child and the Inner Critic, and is more based upon your current experience of life. Your adult self processes more in the moment. While your interpretation of your current experiences are based on the belief systems that were formed by the Inner Child and maintained by the Inner Critic, your adult emotions vacillate more based on external circumstances. For the job ahead, it will take both the thinking part of your adult self as well as its compassionate emotional side. The following steps will guide you in the process.

Step 1: You Must Become Conscious and Believe You Can Change

Make a conscious decision to strengthen your adult self and become conscious of your own thoughts and how they are playing out between the Inner Child and the Inner Critic. Part of this process includes educating yourself as much as possible about how to do this, which of course you are doing with the *Fat to Fearless*® program.

One of the easiest ways to strengthen your adult self is to become more conscious. For your adult self to have power, it has to know that it has power to change the feelings, emotions, and circumstances in your life.

Before you come to know this, you often feel as if you are the victim of your own emotions and external circumstances. This leads to failed attempts to change the circumstances of your life when you focus on the symptoms instead of the root emotional causes.

Focusing on changing the symptoms only leads to a cycle of reinforcing them. However, armed with the knowledge that you are gaining through this book and program, your adult conscious mind knows this is not true and has a way to create positive change in your life.

To do this work, the ultimate belief you must cultivate is the belief that you can change and the past does not equal the future. Your adult self must make a commitment to adopting this belief.

Step 2: Develop an Observer Perspective

Often it is difficult to control your emotions or reactions when you are in the middle of them. During these times, interaction between your Inner Child and Inner Critic are so strong that you easily get lost in the emotion and lose perspective. You believe the way you feel about whatever you are experiencing must be the truth of the situation.

Usually you are vacillating between being dominated by the Inner Critic, internally condemning and criticizing yourself, or giving into the sad, anxious feelings of the Inner Child and letting it engage in whatever behaviors, like eating, it believes will provide relief. These are the times when you need your adult self the most, but have the most trouble accessing it. Cultivating an observer perspective is the quickest and easiest way to access your adult self's resources.

An observer perspective is one in which you pull back from the situation and observe or watch what is going on, especially what is going on in your own head. What thoughts are you thinking, and what pictures are you making in your head? What is the Inner Critic saying, and how is the Inner Child feeling about it?

When you begin asking these questions, you automatically begin moving to an observer's perspective, because the only way to answer them is to take a step back and observe. This also allows you to exercise control over your own state and move from a place of being a victim of your thoughts and feelings to a place of personal empowerment. One of the great things about this shift is that often the act of observing these emotions will minimize the negative emotions and facilitate a positive shift.

Stay in an observer perspective as much as possible. Stay conscious of your thoughts and emotions. React as needed from your adult self to put yourself in as positive a state as possible. You owe this to your Inner Child, because it is your adult self that has made the commitment to reparenting that child and your adult must increase its consciousness to do that.

3. Develop Healthy Assertiveness

Assertiveness is the ability to express yourself openly and honestly and to stand up for your rights and what you know you deserve. Assertiveness is different from aggression. Aggression is based on anger and seeks to win, while assertiveness is based on confidence and seeks a balanced solution that protects your rights while not encroaching on the rights of others.

Assertiveness is important because one of the primary issues is that you have not been sticking up for the wants and needs of your Inner Child. You must learn to assert your rights to protect the Inner Child from both internal criticism and external situations. Every time you don't stand up for yourself you are sending a message straight into your subconscious about what you deserve. Remember, people usually treat us how we have trained them to treat us (which is usually how we have treated our own emotional self).

4. Continue to Use Your Evidence Journal

The adult self needs positive reinforcement. It needs to be reminded of how important it is and all that it brings to the table. It needs to not feel neglected or marginalized. You need to give attention to meeting its needs as well. Providing new opportunities for learning, socialization with other healthy adults, as well as the feelings it gets from being a positive influence on your Inner Child, are all important processes of empowering your adult self.

EXERCISE: CONTEXT SKILLS

One of the principles of Neuro-Linguistic Programming is that many people believe that their abilities are based on context and don't allow skills they have in one area to assist them in others. You may have the belief that losing weight is difficult or the secret fear that you'll always be overweight. Ultimately, at the heart of that is our ability to believe that we can truly choose to make changes and follow through with them.

1. Make a list of all the areas in your life where you have made positive changes and seen those changes through.

2. Now list all of the skills, abilities, and attributes that you have that enabled you to succeed in those areas.

3. Looking at your list, how many of these skills and attributes are you using to help you lose weight? What are the steps you can take to transpose those abilities that you've used to be successful in other areas over to weight loss?

Use your adult self to create a conscious plan to do exactly that. You can even go back to the NLP Reparenting exercise and use the anchoring technique to anchor in those positive attributes. Then when you need them during weight loss challenges, you can fire those anchors and have those skills at the ready. If you decide to do this you may want to use a different physical anchor than the one we used for the previous exercise.

SUMMARY

Key Points

- In the type of reparenting you do as part of the *Fat to Fearless*® program, your adult self will meet the Inner Child's emotional needs, safeguard its interests, and guide it through the process of healing the damage done by the Inner Critic while it learns to believe in your new healthier core beliefs.

- The biggest challenge to reparenting is that a lifetime of ignoring the Inner Child and not defending it against the Inner Critic has led to a lack of trust on the part of the Inner Critic toward your adult self. Meeting its needs consistently, while keeping your word and following through on all of the commitments you make to it, are essential to the process.

- The most important aspect of reparenting your Inner Child is communicating with him/her daily. This can be informal by simply acknowledging and feeling your feelings or formerly using your Inner Child Journal. At this point in your process, I highly recommend using the journal as often as possible until you develop the type of strong connection with this part of you that can be more easily accessed at will.

- Whenever you feel disconnected from your emotions or unable to get in touch with them in a way that allows you to feel better, you are disconnected from your own Inner Child.

- The more we deny and repress our emotions, the more power we give them over us. Eventually, like a beach ball held underwater, they will find a way to the surface.

- Being emotionally whole and complete, which includes feeling all of your feelings and honoring all the parts of yourself, is at the heart of good decision making and healthy intuition.

- As a child, when you determined it was wrong to feel a particular emotion, your Inner Critic, which was responsible for keeping you "right," took over to help you repress and deny those emotions. Often this process of repression and denial becomes automatic—we don't even know what we're not feeling, and frequently these denied feelings show up in the body in the form of obesity and disease.

- Allowing your Inner Child (your emotional self) to fully feel all emotions without negative judgment is integral to the process of healing your Inner Child and ending emotional eating.

- Many people judge certain emotions as bad. Emotions aren't bad, yet sometimes the behaviors that come from these emotions when they are unchecked by your adult self can have a negative impact on your life. Usually this happens when these emotions build after being repressed over time. Every emotion serves a positive purpose in the right context. For example, anger can lead to healthy assertiveness.

- Anchoring is a Neuro-Linguistic Programming technique that associates emotional states with gestures, touches, or sounds that enable these emotional states to be recalled at will by consciously doing the gesture, applying the touch, or hearing the sound. It conditions your brain to fire a response to a chosen stimulus.

- Anchors are a great way to introduce positive feelings into negative memories, providing the opportunity to confuse the prior neurological associations your brain made between the memory and the negative emotions you typically feel when you recall it. This confusion provides an opportunity to neutralize the negative association and introduce a positive-feeling alternative instead.

- While neutralizing the negative feelings associated with past experiences in which your Inner Child was wounded, you also provide a space for your adult self to step in and provide the healthy parenting you didn't receive in that actual remembered experience. When done repeatedly, this reparents the Inner Child and provides much of the positive programming that was previously missing.

- An Inner Child Day is a great way to send the message to your Inner Child that she/he is important and that you value him/her. It does a lot for building a bridge of trust between you and this subconscious part of yourself while also providing a release from the constant pressures of the adult world that often drive us to unhealthy behaviors by repressing the Inner Child's needs.

- Your adult self is the part of you that has made the commitment to reparent your Inner Child. To do that, your adult often needs to be strengthened.

- Developing an observer perspective while also learning healthy assertiveness are important parts of strengthening your adult self.

- The ultimate belief that your conscious mind must choose to adopt to be successful with the *Fat to Fearless*® program or any other major life goal is the belief that you can change and the past does not equal the future.

What This Has To Do With Weight Loss

Emotional eating is undoubtedly the downfall of most people suffering from chronic obesity and weight problems. The emotions that drive you to eat are the results of what your Inner Child feels in response to the self-degradation of the Inner Critic. Ultimately, the Inner Critic just reinforces your negative core beliefs, which are actually the beliefs of your Inner Child.

To change the negative emotions that drive you to overeat, you must change the feelings of the Inner Child. Changing those emotions requires changing its negative beliefs by providing new positive experiences that counteract them with healthier alternatives. All of the exercises in the program do exactly that. However, while changing these negative core beliefs into positive ones, it helps to be able to directly confront and change the negative emotions you are feeling in the moment that are making you crave food. Directly making contact with the Inner Child during these moments by using the techniques in this chapter will allow you to do that and avert episodes of emotional eating.

While some of these exercises are very simple and others seem more complicated, taking the time to do each of them and giving yourself the space and time to allow them to change your subconscious core beliefs will not only change your body but your life as well.

You Are Ready To Move To The Next Chapter When . . .

- You have given yourself at least a week (a month is advised) of doing these exercises daily while continuing to listen to your *Fat to Fearless*® Hypnotherapy Audio Sessions.

- You have watched the tutorial video for this chapter (if you have the full *Fat to Fearless*® program).

- You have completed the exercises for this chapter in the Success Guide and Workbook (if you have the full *Fat to Fearless*® program).

CHAPTER 21

MANAGING PAIN AND PLEASURE

At this point, you have learned a lot about food and emotion. You have learned that emotional self-soothing is behind your poor eating habits that lead to being overweight. You have learned that much of your need to emotionally self-soothe is based on the Inner Critic criticizing the Inner Child. You have also begun the process of transforming the voice of the Inner Critic into a more positive voice while healing the emotional wounds of the Inner Child.

In short, you are finding new ways, other than food, to emotionally satisfy your Inner Child. Now you will learn about the day-to-day management of your levels of pleasure and pain while further releasing your need to emotionally self-soothe with food. You will learn how pain and pleasure specifically relate to emotional eating on a day-to-day basis.

Even after you disempower your Inner Critic and beginning the process of healing, your Inner Child, like all children, will still crave pleasure. Part of that craving for pleasure comes from trying to feel better after a lifetime of being beaten up by the Inner Critic. Healing does not happen overnight. Also, your Inner Child lives in the now and wants to do what feels good in the moment.

Failure to understand this, as well as ensure you have more pleasure than pain in your life on a daily basis, is what leads to breaking down and binging after an otherwise successful period of healthy eating. For our purposes, pain is anything that you don't enjoy doing, as well as the act of denying yourself something you want. When you gain understanding of how pain and pleasure work together to drive you to overeat and learn to make a daily plan to balance these two powerful forces in your life, you will prevent this from happening.

The Inner Child (your emotional self) requires a certain amount of ongoing pleasure. Repressing this need is often the cause of acting out, whether through food, alcohol, sex, drug use, or any other activity that provides the immediate pleasure fix. This acting out also increases in direct relationship to the amount of perceived emotional pain you are feeling. This is why going from one extreme to the other while dieting rarely works and also helps to explain the yo-yo dieting cycle. While writing this book, I experienced a first-hand example of this in my own life.

Finishing the manuscript for this book was one of the busiest and most hectic periods of my life. I had a very busy and successful therapy practice with a full client load, I was writing two books simultaneously, and was also preparing for multiple photo and video shoots. To look my best in these photos and videos, I had increased my workouts as well as become even stricter with my nutrition. I had very little free time and very little pleasure in my life.

I was able to deal with my growing need for pleasure in the moment by focusing on the future payoffs of my efforts. I knew that I could only do this for a limited time and that it was important that I keep the level of pain reasonable, while also making sure I gave my Inner Child enough pleasure to keep it satisfied in the short-term. I was very conscientious of this until I was unexpectedly asked to start teaching hypnotherapy classes on the weekends.

In my capacity as an ACHE Certified Instructor and Examiner, I taught clinical hypnotherapy courses that enabled students to graduate with state-licensed diplomas in hypnotherapy. While I enjoyed working with students in a live class setting, much of the teaching at this school was done through a distance learning system where I was alone in a room with a camera, broadcasting to students around the country.

As a therapist with my specific credentials, all of my training—and my very way of being—is about being fully present with the person in front of me, while reading everything from body language to voice tempo and tone to best understand not only what they are telling me, but what's also going on beneath the surface. Being alone in a room for several hours at a time with only a camera was something I was not accustomed to. In addition to not being well suited for the camera-based teaching system, my work involves the integration of several advanced methods and modalities into an integrated approach, none of which I was able to teach within the classical hypnotherapy curriculum of the school. While it was a good school for those seeking classical hypnotherapy training, the limited educational scope often made teaching frustrating for me.

I had stopped teaching months earlier to focus on the growth of my private practice and the development of the *Fat to Fearless*® program, but a shortage of qualified instructors had the school asking me to step in and teach on a temporary basis. Out of loyalty to the profession, I agreed to teach another six months. This dramatically upset the delicate pain/pleasure balance I was maintaining at the time.

During this time, because of everything in which I was involved, I had no more than half a day on the weekends to spend doing something I enjoyed. This was the time I gave to my Inner Child in exchange for his cooperation in allowing me to be so diligently focused Monday through Saturday.

Teaching meant not only giving up this time but also replacing it with something I didn't enjoy doing for the reasons previously mentioned. I dramatically increased my pain, while decreasing—often eliminating altogether—the only time I had for myself to give my Inner Child the pleasure it desperately needed.

This became an unmanageable equation that before long had me using food on the weekends after teaching to feel better. I quickly realized what was going on and how to change it, and so will you by the time you finish this book and complete the worksheets. I knew I had to decrease my pain and increase my pleasure to avoid turning to food.

I talked to the instructor with whom I was co-teaching the class about changing our schedules. At the time, we worked different days and taught over eight hours on each of our given days. By the end of each day, after talking several hours straight and answering student questions, we were depleted emotionally, mentally, and physically.

We changed the schedule so that instead of having one whole day off after teaching, which was usually spent in a total state of self-soothing to recover before beginning to see clients again on Monday, we would both teach both days with each of us teaching only half of a day. This created a situation where we were not totally drained at the end of each day and we each had two half days to relax and do something pleasurable on the weekend. This restored the pain/pleasure balance, and I immediately stopped turning to food to feel good.

Traditional diets and exercise programs have you plan what you eat, when you eat, how much you eat, and many details related to your fitness program. Yet, without addressing the mind, including the pain/pleasure balance, all of these efforts are doomed to failure. You should spend as much time planning your fitness and diet program as you spend understanding and planning for your daily pain/pleasure balance. This allows you to avoid creating an emotional deficit that overcomes willpower and has you turning to food to compensate.

Part of your ability to do this is going to require you developing alternative sources of pleasure other than food. Most of my clients over the years, and myself when I was overweight, made food the default pleasure drug. To change that, you must expand your list of options for giving yourself pleasure.

When food is your primary source of pleasure in life you will never be successful with a weight loss approach that requires you to significantly reduce what, or how much, you eat. This is in part because, when food is your primary source of pleasure, the amount of food you need to eat each day to feel good is guaranteed to create an overweight body. Also, the longer you deny yourself pleasure, the stronger the cravings become.

In addition to being your primary source of pleasure, if food is your primary mechanism for dealing with pain, then you have two powerful forces driving you to eat. That's why it's important to ensure that you reduce your pain to a tolerable level while increasing your pleasure by also increasing the number of things other than food you enjoy and get satisfaction from.

My client Arthur was a great example of this principle.

Arthur had been overweight most of his life but had gained an extra 50 pounds during his separation and divorce. Now living alone in a small apartment, having lost most of his friends as well as being so overweight that he shied away from social situations, he felt he was at an all-time low.

To make matters worse, Arthur was a web designer and worked from home. Without colleagues he saw on a daily basis, he frequently would go several days without live human interaction. He was determined to lose weight, become more social, and begin dating again. Unfortunately, Taco Bell conspired against him.

Without friends, romantic companionship, or hobbies that he really received pleasure from, Arthur found that the only thing he looked forward to every day was his daily trip to the Taco Bell a mile down the road. Moreover, since this was his only form of daily pleasure, it took a lot of tacos to feel good enough to compensate for all that he felt was lacking in his life.

Every time Arthur tried to deny himself his tacos he would fail. In addition to changing his negative core beliefs, disempowering his Inner Critic, and healing his Inner Child, I knew Arthur needed to find new sources of pleasure besides food or he would never be successful in losing weight and keeping it off.

Despite his reluctance, I was able to get Arthur to develop a hobby, and begin socializing and making new friends. Quickly, not only was he getting pleasure from things other than food, but he also had more motivation to lose weight as new dating possibilities entered his life. While we still had a lot of work to do, ultimately no amount of Inner Child work or changing core beliefs was going to allow him to lose weight until he found pleasure in something other than food and ensured he had an adequate amount of that pleasure to keep him from running for the border at the end of each day.

Lastly, part of what kept Arthur from "getting out more" was his fear and shame around his body. Dealing with this was also instrumental in allowing him to experience more pleasure in other areas of his life. We will be working on this directly in the last exercise of the *Fat to Fearless*® program.

Your first step in the process of tipping your daily pleasure/ pain balance toward enabling weight loss is for you to become conscious of where you are at now on the scale and then make a plan to make sure you have the right amount of pleasure in your life in proportion to your level of pain. By doing this, you will ensure you don't have a pleasure deficit that has you reaching for food. If you have the *Fat to Fearless*® Success Guide and Workbook, turn to the worksheets for this section. If not, instructions are below:

EXERCISE: BALANCING PAIN AND PLEASURE

1. Begin keeping a daily pleasure/pain index log. Write down all of your activities for the day, leaving a margin to the right of each activity where you can rate it on the pain/ pleasure scale. This might include the hours you spend

working in front of the computer, lunch with a colleague, running errands, watching TV, eating dinner, etc.

2. Rate each activity using the following scale:

> 5: I Love This!
>
> 4: Highly Enjoyable
>
> 3: Enjoyable
>
> 2: Slightly Pleasurable
>
> 1: I Don't Mind It
>
> 0: Neutral, Take it or Leave it
>
> -1: Rather Not Do It
>
> -2: Slightly Unpleasant
>
> -3: Unpleasant
>
> -4: Highly Unpleasant
>
> -5: Absolutely Hate This!

3. Now on a scale from 0 to 10, with 0 being "Not At All" and 10 being "Intense Need and Urge," write down where you would rate your desire each day to eat foods and/or quantities of foods not in keeping with your weight loss eating plan.

4. Notice the correlation between these two numbers. If you want the desire to overeat or eat the wrong foods to go down, then you must increase your overall pleasure number for the day (not using food!). You must give your Inner Child more joy to keep it from turning to food.

5. Make an active plan to add more enjoyable activities, reduce unenjoyable activities, or make the less enjoyable activities more enjoyable until your pleasure number is at the point where your urges to emotionally eat are manageable.

*For many, cravings can feel like an uncontrollable urge that leaves little time to act mindfully before they find themselves indulging in unhealthy pleasures. If this is you, get more information on how to quickly stop cravings in the moment at the following webpage:

www.asherfoxweightloss.com/stopcravings

SUMMARY

Key Points

- Your Inner Child (your emotional self) requires a certain amount of pleasure each day. Not having the adequate amount of pleasure each day is often what causes us to turn to food to compensate. We've learned from a lifetime of experience that food provides quick pleasure and restores our daily "feel good" tank (at least in the very short term).

- The longer you deny yourself pleasure, the more that need builds until eventually you give in. Binge-eating is a frequent release for not having enough enjoyment in your life. The longer you've lived in denial, the greater the binge.

- Overly restrictive diets fail in part because they take away too much of the one thing you've learned to turn to for pleasure, which is food.

- For our purposes, pain is anything you don't enjoy doing as well as the act of denying yourself something you want. The greater the amount of pain in your life, both daily and cumulatively, the more pleasure you need to offset that pain.

- You should spend as much time planning the amount of pleasure and pain you experience as you do planning your nutrition and exercise to ensure you're not turning to food to compensate for lack of pleasure.

- Increasing the number of activities that you can get pleasure from instead of food will be important to balance your daily pain/pleasure to avoid emotional eating.

- Using your *Fat to Fearless*® Success Guide and Workbook you can become conscious of your daily pleasure/pain score and correlate it to your desire to overeat. When you know your pain/pleasure score, you can make a conscious plan to reduce your pain, increase your pleasure, and decrease your desire to emotionally eat.

What This Has To Do With Weight Loss

If you don't ensure you are getting more pleasure than pain on a daily basis, you will turn to food to balance the scales (pun intended). Ultimately, the basic drive to move away from pain and toward pleasure overrides everything else. Without learning to find pleasure from things other than food and making sure you have enough of that pleasure while working to reduce "pain" as much as possible, emotional eating will always be a problem for those with lifelong chronic weight issues.

You Are Ready To Move To The Next Chapter When . . .

- You have watched the tutorial video for this chapter (if you have the full *Fat to Fearless*® program).

- You have completed the exercises for this chapter in the Success Guide and Workbook (if you have the full *Fat to Fearless*® program).

PART VI

LIVING FEARLESSLY

ARE YOU READY?

I n this section you will begin your final steps on your *Fat to Fearless*® journey, which are the first steps toward actually living life fearlessly. If you've followed the program up to this point and have done all of the exercises for each of the chapters and sections, while giving yourself and your subconscious mind the time to transform, change, and accept new programming—then you are in a dramatically different place than when you started. The quickest you should've gone through the program to reach this point is 8 weeks, with many taking a full 12 to 24 weeks. This is the time required to ensure you've followed the instructions for listening to all of the Hypnotherapy Audio Sessions and learned your new skills, while taking the time to actively apply them to allow the necessary changes to take place at the subconscious level. Before you move into the final part of the program, *Living Fearlessly*, let's review what you've learned so far.

- You have learned about the power of the subconscious mind and how, in conjunction with your core beliefs, it has caused you to self-sabotage all of your past dieting efforts.

- You've uncovered your own specific core beliefs as well as chosen and begun installing new more positive core beliefs that will support you in achieving permanent weight loss.

- You've learned about your Inner Critic and how to disarm it by spotting its cognitive distortions as well as learning to use the power of humor and your own personalized affirmations.

- You've learned how the Inner Critic—in conjunction with your R.A.S. and Critical Gateway—preserves your existing core beliefs and makes it difficult to change them without specific techniques and hypnotherapy audios based on unique methodologies like the ones in this program. As you've gone through the program, you've learned how to make the three mechanisms of the subconscious mind work for you, instead of against you. They now preserve your new more positive core beliefs in the way they previously preserved your negative ones.

- You've learned about and developed a relationship with your Inner Child, which is your emotional self. You've come to understand how the negative feelings that cause you to overeat emanate from this part of you. You've also begun helping your Inner Child heal from childhood wounds and negative beliefs through reparenting it, so it no longer needs to turn to food to feel good.

- You've come to understand the importance of balancing pain and pleasure on a daily basis to ensure you don't try to make up that pleasure deficit with food.

As a result of the above—assuming you've been listening to your Hypnotherapy Audio Sessions throughout the program—you should now notice the following changes:

You can now easily see how your entire life up to this point, including your prior inability to lose weight and keep it off, has been a result of your subconscious mind acting to prove your negative core beliefs to be true. Because of this, when you find yourself engaging in old behaviors and thought patterns, you're able to easily identify past programming and use the techniques you've learned to put yourself back on the path toward achieving your goals. You find that the more you do this, the less often it happens, and the easier it gets.

Because you understand that the subconscious mind is influenced by repetition and emotion, you are constantly programming yourself for weight loss success through the use of your affirmations and your Hypnotherapy Audio Sessions.

You notice your Inner Critic is much less active and has much less influence on your life. When it does begin its criticism, you immediately identify its cognitive distortions, apply challenge questions, and minimize its power by using submodality changes (reducing the volume, pitch, and tone), while also using humor and fighting back with your positive affirmations. You find that the more time that goes by, the less power it has, and the more it seems to be transforming into a less negative voice.

You're much more in touch with your emotional self (Inner Child) and are learning to love all of yourself, especially the emotions you used to judge and repress. Part of learning to love yourself has been learning to assertively stand up for your Inner Child and ensure it knows it's loved and valued just as it is. You've also identified ways of providing healthy pleasure to your Inner Child, so it doesn't always need food to feel better and actively give yourself and your Inner Child those forms of healthy enjoyment.

You are actively working to ensure you have more pleasure than pain in your life so you don't need to turn to food to overcome a deficit of emotional pleasure. You also have stopped severe deprivation dieting because you realize it only leads to a rebound effect where you eventually make up that pleasure through long periods of unhealthy or binge eating.

Overall, you should find your self-esteem has dramatically increased, continues to do so, and you have a much deeper understanding of yourself than ever before.

If the above statements describe the changes you've experienced going through the *Fat to Fearless*® program, then you're ready to move forward to the final step. If you feel like you're still dramatically struggling with what I've described above, I would suggest going back through the program from the beginning, taking more time to do the exercises, and allowing yourself the time to fully experience each subconscious and emotional change before moving on to the next chapter. Also, I would recommend joining one of my online coaching groups so you can have more one-on-one guidance directly from me as you go through the process. You can get more information on joining a *Fat to Fearless*® online coaching program at: asherfoxweightloss.com/groupcoaching.

It is important to understand that this type of deep and powerful change is progressive and gradual. When reading the list above you shouldn't have the expectation that you're 100% in all of them, or even in any one. We are always changing and improving as long as were living and moving forward; going from *Fat to Fearless*® is very much about the journey and not the destination. That doesn't mean that the destination, if defined as your goal weight, is unimportant. What it means is that as long as that number on the scale is all that matters and you define your self-worth by it, then you will never love yourself enough to engage in the behavior that helps you reach that healthy weight. It also means you have to wait until you reach that goal to value yourself enough to begin living life fully and fearlessly.

If you feel ready to move on to the last section of the *Fat to Fearless*® program, it is time for you to learn about and overcome secondary gains. Beyond proving your negative core beliefs to be true, your subconscious may actually believe you are actually better off being overweight.

Bypassing secondary gains is one of the final steps in the *Fat to Fearless*® process because to do so requires you having learned the skills involved in, and actively already worked on, resolving your negative core beliefs and replacing them with positive ones, disempowering your Inner Critic, healing and loving your Inner Child, and adopting the belief that you can produce deep changes in your inner life that will subsequently be reflected in your outer life.

Let's get started.

CHAPTER 22

MOTIVATIONS: SEEN AND UNSEEN

What positive benefit do you get from being overweight? At first, this question may seem absurd, but the answer is important to understand because it is the last piece of the puzzle as to why you have unsuccessfully tried so hard for so long to lose weight. It's time to learn what subconscious and hidden motivation you have for staying overweight and what you can do to change that motivation.

Over the years, I have learned to ask one very simple question of my clients to help them become open to this concept. I ask them to rate on a scale of 1 to 10 how important it is to them to lose weight and achieve the body they want. Most answer with a 9 or 10.

I then spend time discussing their answer to make sure it is accurate. I review the list of things that are usually more important, such as their children and family. After more discussion, their weight loss goals usually end up around a realistic 8, but rarely go below a 7.

Then comes the important question. I say something like this: "You seem to be an intelligent and capable person. You have managed to support yourself all these years by holding a job, gained the skills and education necessary for that job, and have overcome many obstacles, many of which required great willpower and follow-through, to have all of the things you currently have in your life. How can something be an 8 in importance to you throughout most of your life, and yet you not have achieved it—unless there is something you are unaware of standing in your way?"

This simple realization opens the door for most to accept that there is something much deeper going on. They begin to consider the possibility that they get something out of being overweight of which they are not aware.

Some people tell me they know what has gotten in the way: *They love food, and they do not like exercise.* While this may be true, I point out there are lots of things they have accomplished even though they would rather be doing something else and do not like the activities involved.

For example, you may have enjoyed partying and hated studying, yet you still managed to get through school. At this point, I usually have their attention, and I introduce them to the concept of primary and secondary gains.

Primary and secondary gains are the direct and indirect advantages a person receives from maintaining a particular state, condition, or behavior. The direct advantage, which is often the motivator for beginning the behavior, is called the primary gain.

The indirect advantage, which usually becomes the stronger subconscious motivation for keeping the behavior over time, is the secondary gain. While most people are consciously aware of the primary gain, the secondary gain usually remains hidden to the person. Let's look at some examples to illustrate the concept.

A smoker often began smoking at a young age to fit in with a particular peer group. This is the primary reason he began smoking, and even if he will not admit to it, he is usually aware that this is why he is doing it. This is the primary gain, and he is aware of the benefit he gets from the behavior. Over time, smoking and the associated chemicals become a means of dealing with stressful situations and allows him to repress and not deal with painful emotions and situations. While he may be aware to varying degrees that smoking relaxes him, he probably does not realize that it allows him, much like food for an overeater, to avoid dealing with the causes of stress and negative emotions. These are the secondary gains.

Let's look at some other examples.

Sally often feels lonely and depressed and turns to the pleasure rush of sugar to feel better, even when she is not hungry. She is aware of the connection between food and her sad feelings, and knows she eats for emotional reasons. This is the primary gain. Sally also has a strong fear of rejection and avoids dating. Because overeating also causes her to be overweight, her self-image is so poor that she avoids most social activities where she might meet men, which in turn keeps her from putting herself in situations that might eventually lead to the rejection she fears. She is unaware of this connection, which makes it all the more powerful in her life. The secondary gain for Sally to being overweight is that it protects her from rejection.

Jill provides another example beyond weight issues:

Jill was grateful to be a cancer survivor. Over the past few years, she had triumphed over her illness with the help and support of her family and friends. Far longer than she knew was necessary, she sheltered herself from re-engaging in life, largely because she liked the attention she received from friends who came to spend time with her because she was still "recovering." Before her illness, some of her closest family and friends rarely made the time to drive from the city to her suburban home.

She knows on some level that she is better than she leads everyone to believe. She is even aware she is slowing her own recovery because she likes the company. The attention she gets is the primary gain received from re-engaging life. But there is more to this story.

Before leaving work to begin treatment, she felt her performance slipping, and it seemed to be reflected in her supervisors' attitudes toward her work. She began to doubt she was any good at what she did and feared what that meant for her future. What Sally didn't realize was that by taking longer to recover than was necessary, she was able to continue telling herself she was excellent at what she did and just had a couple of bad months. For Sally, avoiding the fear of finding out she "wasn't good enough" at work was the secondary gain to her prolonging her recovery.

Now that you understand the concept of primary and secondary gains, let's look more deeply at primary gains.

As you have already learned, primary gains are the direct benefit of engaging in a behavior and the person is usually aware this is why they do it. Almost every overweight person knows the pleasure that comes from food. We've called it emotional self-soothing, and this is almost always the primary gain of overeating. The best way to deal with the primary gain of emotional eating is to address the root cause: the emotions and the negative core beliefs behind them. Addressing these emotions is what you have learned to do up to this point by:

1. Working to change your negative core beliefs into positive ones.

2. Healing your Inner Child (emotional self) while disempowering the Inner Critic.

3. Monitoring, managing, and planning your level of pleasure and pain each day to ensure you have less "pain" and more pleasure so that you don't turn to food to make up the deficit.

Sometimes though it's not always the "happy chemicals" produced by the food itself but other byproducts of unhealthy eating that are the primary gains. Let's look at a few of those now.

Social Bonding

Food is central to most social activities. Many people are aware of this and avoid social gatherings when they are on a diet. The challenge is that a lack of social activity can lead to feelings of isolation and sadness that then lead to using food to feel better.

Food often has the effect of making you feel connected. What most people don't realize is this feeling of connection is a projection of what you are feeling within yourself, because the pleasure of food bridges the gap between your adult self and the Inner Child. That feeling of internal connection coupled with the initially positive brain chemicals that come from food, specifically sugar, seduces you into engaging in eating behaviors that keep you overweight.

The key to overcoming this primary gain is to become very consciously aware of it. You must consciously place focus on the emotional interactions you have with the people you are socializing with, as opposed to the food. Imagine if your Inner Child received all the pleasure it needed from the joy of socializing (in social situations). Consciously imagine these positive feelings filling up your Inner Child and quenching the emotional needs it would normally turn to food to get. It helps to talk to your Inner Child, so remind it of all of the positive things that come from losing weight. Remind your Inner Child it can feel good from only socializing without also overeating.

Another important component of eliminating this primary gain is learning how to *savor* food. Most people eat more quickly than they can actually taste the food. In one exercise I do with my clients, I give them a piece of chocolate, and I tell them to allow it to dissolve on their tongue. They slowly, fully, and completely enjoy it. I then give them a second piece, and I ask them how it tastes compared to the first piece. They usually report that they taste the second piece of chocolate only half as much as the first.

This is how our taste buds work. Flavor continues to diminish after the first exposure, yet we keep eating as if we are chasing the first bite. Make a conscious effort to take one bite of the food, slowly chew and enjoy it, and then take the second bite and notice the difference in taste. When you become conscious of this, it is easier to sample different dishes at social venues without eating too much of any one thing.

Boredom

While eating to avoid boredom is a form of emotional self-soothing, it needs to be addressed in different ways. One of the issues that many suffer from in our society is feeling a lack of purpose. Instead of meaningful careers, too many of us just have jobs. Instead of passions, we settle for hobbies. If you eat to avoid boredom, ask yourself if you have a life purpose and if there are things you feel passionate about. What activities excite you that you could fill your time with that you previously spent eating?

If you feel you lack purpose in life, there are many books and programs that can help you find your life's calling. In a life where we *only* have 80 to 100 or so years to live, I believe we should never be bored. There is so much to see, do, and accomplish, and when you connect with your life purpose, I know you will passionately feel the same. In comparison to the excitement of living a passionate and purpose-filled life, food can't compete as a tool to alleviate boredom.

Beyond finding a purpose for your life, I could discuss techniques for distracting yourself with other things to stave off boredom, but I won't. In my experience, people who have found their purpose in life are never bored, and I firmly believe that it is the ultimate and only worthwhile solution to overcoming this primary gain. To distract yourself with something else other than food to alleviate boredom is simply replacing one neurosis for another. Find your purpose in life, ignite your passion, and leave boredom behind.

Beyond social bonding and alleviating boredom, there could be other primary gains as well. I had one client who had a crush on a local baker. Every day she would go in and eat several pastries in an attempt to spend time with him. The primary gain here was obvious. The point I want to make is that there can be as many primary gains and secondary gains as there are people, the key is for you to find those that are uniquely yours to begin counteracting them.

Your primary gains are usually fairly easy to spot; it's the secondary gains—the hidden benefits of being overweight that you're not aware of—that present the most problems. In the next chapter we will uncover and defeat these hidden subconscious motivations for staying overweight.

Complete the exercise below in your *Fat to Fearless*® Success Guide and Workbook or on your own paper.

EXERCISE: DIFFUSING PRIMARY GAINS

1. List the main benefits you get from food.

2. Create a conscious plan to get these needs met in other ways. For example:

   If you eat emotionally, we already discussed in the prior chapter on managing pain and pleasure the need to find new activities that you enjoy to replace food. Using the Pain/Pleasure Daily Balance sheets in your *Fat to Fearless*® Success Guide and Workbook, ensure you're getting adequate levels of pleasure from these activities.

   If social bonding is a primary gain, plan social events that don't involve food, such as hiking. Use these events as an opportunity to begin training your brain and Inner Child so you can enjoy socialization without the need to eat.

   If boredom is an issue, make a plan to begin exploring your own wants and needs in an effort to find something that ignites your passion. When you find this, you will rarely be bored as there will always be some activity you can do to support you in this passion.

SUMMARY

Key Points

- Primary and secondary gains are the direct and indirect advantages a person receives from maintaining a particular state, condition, or behavior. For our purposes it can be defined as "what you get out of being overweight."

- If you have been able to graduate from school, support yourself financially, or raise a family and have overcome all of the obstacles to enable you to do that, it only makes sense that if you can't lose weight, there is something you're unaware of holding you back. After all, in all of the above examples, which require a great deal of willpower to follow through, you were able to overcome all of the obstacles that were in your path as you became aware of them. These types of subconscious stumbling blocks typically remain hidden, which is why you haven't been able to directly address them.

- Beyond the obvious immediate gratification of the way food makes us feel, often social bonding and boredom are other primary gains that need to be addressed.

- Learning to savor food is one way to help mitigate overeating during social events. Savoring is a great skill to acquire to help with weight loss.

- Finding a life purpose that ignites your passion ensures there is rarely a time you will feel bored. In addition, being driven by your passion often has additional benefits toward losing weight, as it may create new motivations for being slimmer and healthy.

- Primary gains are usually easily seen and can be dealt with by creating a conscious plan while at the same time continuing your subconscious work that you have been doing throughout the *Fat to Fearless*® program.

What This Has To Do With Weight Loss

All behavior exists because at one point in time, in some context, it served a purpose. Overeating or craving unhealthy foods is a behavior that, to have existed so long throughout your life, must serve a purpose. Typically, there are two purposes: one that is usually known (primary gain) and one that is hidden (secondary gain). Addressing primary gains and uncovering and defeating secondary gains is one of the final steps in your *Fat to Fearless*® journey.

You Are Ready To Move To The Next Chapter When . . .

- You have watched the tutorial video for this chapter (if you have the full *Fat to Fearless*® program).

- You have completed the exercises for this chapter in the Success Guide and Workbook (if you have the full *Fat to Fearless*® program).

CHAPTER 23

UNCOVERING SECONDARY GAINS

Secondary gains is the psychological term for the less-than-obvious and usually unconscious motivations that exert more influence over our behaviors than we might possibly imagine. Because of their hidden nature, which makes them difficult for us to see and address, they often have more of an impact on our lives than their more obvious counterparts: primary gains.

Another reason secondary gains are so difficult to deal with is that we don't want to. If you were willing to deal directly with the issue behind the secondary gain (using weight to avoid intimacy for instance), you would not use indirect behavior to avoid doing so (such as being overweight). Since you are unconsciously trying to not deal with these behaviors, you are invested in not unmasking the secondary gain that manifests through poor eating habits and excess weight because they protect you from what you fear the most. Let us refer back to a previous example.

Sally prolonged her recovery and put off re-engaging life after illness because of the attention she received from her friends and family. This was her primary gain. Her secondary gain was that she did not have to confront the possibility that she was not very good at her job. She was conscious of her primary gain, but the secondary gain was mostly beyond her awareness.

Because of her unwillingness to confront her fears about her career, the secondary gain developed. If she were forced to face this subconscious payoff, it might force her to face her fears, which she is not ready to do. Therefore, she is highly motivated on multiple levels to not acknowledge the secondary gain and risk disarming it in a way that would force her to deal with the true issue at hand. Secondary gains are often a powerful denial mechanism and as such function very effectively beneath the surface. Nowhere is this more true than in weight loss. The following case study from my client Judy is a great example.

Judy came to see me 2 years after her husband's death—and 60 pounds heavier. Her husband had left her well provided for, and she had spent the past two years filling her time with community outreach projects, political fundraisers, and her dog, Joe. She struggled with her weight most of her life, engaging in the common yo-yo cycle, yet it had become much worse since her husband's death, and she did not understand why.

While she had certainly gone through a grieving process, she considered that to be far behind her. While her husband had been a good man, they did not have a passionate marriage. In truth, she questioned whether they ever really loved each other. She appreciated that he had provided well for her during his lifetime and had left her well taken care of, but she didn't consider her life before his death any better than her life now. In many ways, she preferred her single status and the freedom that came with it.

She spent much of this newfound freedom in solitude with her dog, Joe. She dated very little since being widowed, yet when she came to see me, she had been in a relationship for about three months. She believed he was not any more serious about her than she was about him, which was not that serious at all. He was someone to do things with casually.

Her weight issues were caused less by lack of exercise than by her eating habits. As a matter of fact, she exercised religiously at least three times a week, yet found that the harder she exercised, the more she sabotaged herself with her diet. Her yo-yo cycle was more extreme than most, consisting of almost starving herself every other day while gorging herself on the alternate days. She would eat well past the point of being full until she felt actual physical pain in her stomach. She came to me to find out why.

While I had managed to reduce her overeating and binge yo-yo cycle dramatically in the first two sessions, it was in the third session that the big breakthrough came. Using her feelings around the symptoms (out-of-control eating), I did a hypnotherapeutic age regression and uncovered the associated beliefs and the events that led to them.

Starting around age five, she had multiple experiences with her father that led her to believe he preferred her sister and did not love her. From these events she formed the belief that if anyone got to know her they would find out she was not good enough and would not like her.

Throughout the years, she developed a variety of coping mechanisms designed to keep her from getting close to people in an effort to avoid the pain of confirming her negative subconscious core beliefs. She didn't want them to find out that she was flawed, and then reject her in the way that small child believed her father had. She had even managed to marry a man who was as distant as she was, traveled for much of their marriage, and seemed to have little interest in getting to know the real her.

Even in her marriage, she avoided rejection by avoiding intimacy. After her husband's death, her extra pounds were another way of continuing that trend. Because she was so self-conscious about her appearance, she rarely went to social functions. She assumed that men she might actually be interested in on a deeper level would not be interested in her if they spent too much time with her.

The primary gain of her binge eating was the emotional self-soothing that came from food, specifically the same type of sweets her mother gave her whenever she was feeling sad or rejected as a child. In hypnosis, she was clearly able to tell me she ate to the point of literal stomach pain because she was trying to fill the emptiness inside that came from a lifetime of no intimacy with others. She also had no intimate relationship with her own inner self since she had spent the same lifetime repressing these emotions and being disconnected from her Inner Child. Binge eating, which temporarily satisfied the pain of her Inner Child, was the closest she ever came to feeling connected with that child, to feeling connected to herself.

The secondary gain was that as long as she was overweight she would never feel good enough about her body to engage others to the point that they might get to know her well enough to reject her.

Using the same methods taught through the *Fat to Fearless*® program, she was able to change this core belief. She began to know others more closely and eventually learned to fill her void with intimacy instead of with food. With diligent work and time, she eliminated both the primary and secondary gains associated with her eating behavior.

The last time I checked in with Judy she had reached her goal weight and was in a happy relationship with a man she had met through a fundraising event.

In the above example, you can see how Judy was aware that the primary gain from overeating was emotional self-soothing. She did not quite understand fully what she was trying to soothe—lack of intimacy—because she had repressed it and denied the conscious need for it. But she did know she ate to feel better. She was unaware of the secondary gain because she was unwilling to even admit she had such a fear of closeness with others or that she had the negative core beliefs that drove that fear.

It would have been very unlikely she could have made the connection on her own through the process of simply living her life. Even if she had been able to, without the tools to change those beliefs and heal her emotional self, her fears would have kept her from wanting to acknowledge them. This is why it is so important in this process to uncover your negative core beliefs and their associated secondary gains. They work together to keep you in the dark about your own deep inner self so you continuously construct a life and body consistent with these limiting childhood beliefs.

Krissy's story is a great example of the power of secondary gains to sabotage weight loss efforts even in the face of severe medical issues caused by morbid obesity.

I started working with Krissy about 15 years ago, and she was one of my first severely obese clients. She had been referred to me by her physician with a prognosis of less than two years to live without a dramatic reduction in her weight. Standing 5-feet-tall, she weighed over 450 pounds and was barely mobile.

Our first meeting was a dramatic one. She sobbed in my office while telling me that she would do anything to lose weight, not just because she desperately wanted to live, but also because of how miserable her very existence had become. Not only was she barely able to walk, but she also had trouble taking care of basic personal hygiene to the point that she'd been isolated away from all of the other workers at her office because they had complained of the smell. She hated her life and told me that she would do anything to change.

My heart went out to her, and I decided I would do whatever it took to help her. At this point in my career, I was not only dealing with the psychological and emotional issues of my clients, but as a Certified Medical Exercise Specialist, was also supervising most of their fitness and nutrition programs. She promised to do her part, and we began treatment.

By her third session, she was showing improvement in her mobility from her exercises and told me she was compliant with her nutrition. She felt slightly better physically, but emotionally she felt much better because for the first time she had hope and felt like she had found someone that could truly help her. I was elated that I was making such a difference in her life and was looking forward to beginning to work on more of the psychological and emotional issues around her weight. I didn't anticipate what happened next.

About three weeks into her program, I was having lunch with a colleague at a Subway restaurant that was across the street from both a Burger King and McDonald's. I saw her car pull into the McDonald's drive-in. I knew it was her car because I not only could see her through the window, but it also severely listed to one side because of her weight. I watched as three bags were handed to her from the McDonald's drive-thru, and she then drove to the Burger King drive-thru where she received another bag of food.

The colleague I was with had been a part of the intake and medical referral process when she came to our clinic, and she knew about her case history. She told me I should drop her as a client because she obviously wasn't serious about losing weight and didn't care about her health. Although I was taken aback by what I had just witnessed, I remembered the sincerity behind the pleas for help in my office a few weeks earlier and knew that there had to be something much deeper going on.

It did not take long for me to learn through our sessions why, no matter how great the consequences of her excess weight and no matter how great her conscious effort to lose the weight, she continued to sabotage herself in the worst possible ways. As a child, she had been repeatedly molested and raped by a family member she trusted. Although she did not make the conscious connection, it was the driving force behind her severe obesity. Her weight was her protection against ever being raped or touched against her will again. As long as she was morbidly obese and believed herself to be unattractive, she subconsciously believed she was safe from the attention of men.

In this instance, the secondary gain was linked directly to her survival instinct, which made it impossible for her subconscious to allow her to lose weight until it was resolved. Her obesity was also a matter of survival since she'd been given a prognosis of death within the next two years if she didn't lose weight. However, if you remember from your primer on the mind at the beginning of this book, the subconscious acts upon what is known to it. Being told that she would die of obesity within a couple of years was an intellectual concept, something to process in the conscious mind, and not based on past experience. However, while she had never died from obesity before, she most certainly had the experience of being molested and raped when she was thin. To the subconscious, what has happened before and what is known is acted upon as fact. This was a fact that her subconscious believed needed to be acted upon to protect her by keeping her overweight and undesirable.

Just like before, we see the primary gain, of which she was conscious, was using food to ease her loneliness and depression. The secondary gain, which she did not consciously realize, was to keep her safe and protect her from being violated. While it took some time, we eventually resolved this for her in a way that allowed her to make significant weight loss progress.

My former client Frank presents another example of an inability to lose weight because of secondary gains.

Frank was a divorced father of three with full-time custody of his children. After getting married, it became apparent that his wife had significant emotional issues he'd been unaware of when they were dating. Shortly after the birth of their children she left, saying she couldn't deal with the pressure of being a wife and a mother. Outside of an occasional letter with no return address, she had not been in contact with the family for years.

Frank was almost 50 and about 100 pounds overweight. He would try to diet and exercise, but as soon as he began making progress, he would binge to where he not only regained what he had lost, but several extra pounds as well. In a hypnotherapy session, I spoke directly to the part of him that was overeating and through that dialogue came to understand what was going on.

Frank had the subconscious belief that he was at fault for his wife leaving and his family falling apart. He felt he needed to make up for that by being the best possible father. He also believed that being the best father meant giving 100% of his time and emotional energy to his children. When he started taking time to exercise and attend to his own health, he subconsciously believed it was taking time away from his family. He thought that others who saw him exercising and looking better would think he was an irresponsible and selfish parent for focusing on his own needs.

In hypnosis, he revealed that being a good father was the only thing he felt he had left to do right in his life, and that it was more important than his own health. Once this belief became conscious, Frank consciously decided it was true, that being a good father meant taking no time for himself. He decided it would be irresponsible of him to exercise or plan his meals or not have candy, cakes, and snacks around all the time that the kids wanted, even though they were also becoming overweight. Frank opted to not deal with his secondary gain after it was uncovered, and the last I checked, he was now more than 150 pounds overweight.

Frank's story is an excellent example of the forces we must be willing to tackle if we are to defeat our secondary gains. As I stated earlier, secondary gains are a means of not dealing directly with what the true underlying issue is. Our unwillingness to face these issues perpetuates our inability to acknowledge and tear down our hidden motivations to remaining overweight. This is also a great example of the role our adult self must play in this process.

It is our adult self that, once these hidden motivations and the negative core beliefs that spawned them are unmasked, must choose to reject them in favor of healthier perspectives and better means of dealing with our daily lives. In Frank's case, his adult self (his conscious mind) chose to accept the belief that spending time taking care of his own needs made him a bad parent. Remember from our section on strengthening your adult self that it is our conscious mind (our adult self) that must choose to adopt the belief that change is possible, and then choose to engage in the activities to create that change. Frank chose not to do that and subsequently is still overweight.

To achieve permanent weight loss, your secondary gains must be unmasked, and the related unhealthy core beliefs and the fears surrounding them must be dealt with. All of these mechanisms that keep you overweight are a direct reflection of your negative core beliefs, the same ones you are now in the process of changing into new healthier beliefs.

Below are some of the most common secondary gains that keep people from losing weight. I have personally encountered all of these numerous times in my almost 20 years of helping clients. As you read these, see if any of them resonate with you. While you may be consciously unaware that you have some of these secondary gains, frequently (but not always) your body will give you clues to the ones you are not conscious of. Note any of these that cause you any feeling of dis-ease or physical or emotional discomfort.

COMMON SECONDARY GAINS PREVENTING PERMANENT WEIGHT LOSS

Emotions Brought Up by Attention From the Opposite Sex

Although you believe you want to be more attractive by losing weight, often that attractiveness is something you are emotionally unprepared for. If you have never received a lot of attention from the opposite sex, then it is usually accompanied by feelings of being uncomfortable, vulnerable, awkward, and sometimes even unsafe. Additionally, this type of attention brings up the possibility of physical intimacy, which can bring up any issues you have related to sex. Time and again I have seen people achieve considerable weight loss only to begin self-sabotaging themselves when they start getting the attention they thought they craved.

Negative Core Beliefs: Frequently the attached core beliefs are related to "not being good enough," being "unlovable," being "unattractive/ugly," "I'm not safe," or "sex is bad." These core beliefs often are coupled with other beliefs such as "all men cheat," "relationships mean loss of freedom," and so on.

Avoiding Finding Out If You Are "Good Enough"

This is one of the most powerful secondary gains that remains hidden because of its lack of obviousness. If you have chronic weight problems, your dreams are often directly connected to the vision you have of yourself with a better body. Sometimes that is your whole dream.

Usually, however, part of the dream is what you will do once you have the body you want. You will date more, have the confidence to start that new business, do public presentations, be taken more seriously at work, and maybe even follow that dream of dance lessons and doing dance competitions. You will get out more, do more, and *live life more fearlessly.* These are but a few of what many people plan for their future life with their new body.

You consciously believe that you have what it takes to do all of these things, but your weight has been what is holding you back. You consciously believe that once the weight is gone, the world is yours. However, your conscious beliefs about your capabilities may be at odds with your subconscious negative core beliefs.

The challenge comes when the negative core beliefs that sabotage your weight loss efforts also permeate your other dreams. For instance, the core belief that "I'm not good enough" or "I'm unlovable," not only sabotages your weight loss efforts but also undermines your future goals independent of the shape of your body as well.

You are able to consciously tell yourself that you can do these things because as long as you are overweight, you do not have to risk finding out that maybe you can't. As you lose weight, the reality of doing them sets in and the subconscious fear that you may not be good enough to do them causes you to self-sabotage your weight loss efforts. As long as you stay overweight and make losing weight a prerequisite for doing these things, you don't have to risk finding out that you can't accomplish those goals because you are in some way not capable or not good enough regardless of how you physically look and feel.

Negative Core Beliefs: This secondary gain can be attached to almost all of your limiting beliefs about yourself. "I'm not good enough" in some form is almost always present.

Not Becoming What You Resent

A fundamental rule of the subconscious is that you can't become what you resent. In weight loss, I have seen this with clients who judge people that have a healthy weight as getting an unfair advantage and getting ahead because of it. I have known many women who resent female coworkers they consider thin and attractive. They believe the success of these women they consider more attractive than themselves is because of their physical appearance and firmly believe they do not want to be one of those women. As long as they have this judgment, they subconsciously deny themselves the bodies they equate to this concept. The secondary gain to being overweight is a combination of avoiding becoming what they resent and the feeling of believing their accomplishments aren't based on how they look. Subconsciously, it is more important to them to feel as if their achievements aren't based on appearance or how thin they are than it is to lose weight. Resolving this secondary gain is critical to long-term weight loss success.

Negative Core Beliefs: Core beliefs linked to this secondary gain tend to be very specific and individual, based on what aspects are resented and judged in self and others.

Weight As a Safety Mechanism

While weight can be a defense mechanism against attention from the opposite sex, it can also be powerfully rooted in basic safety and survival. This is often the case in instances of childhood sexual abuse or forced or coerced sex at any age. The idea is that being overweight makes the person unattractive to the opposite sex and diminishes the likelihood they will be a target.

In my experience, when this is the root secondary gain, it is most frequently manifested as excessive obesity. It is important to not make a generalization that this is the case for all people who fall into this weight category as there can be many other causes. When this is the case, however, healing the negative core beliefs that came from the event are critical to resolving the secondary gain. This is absolutely necessary before weight loss can be achieved. This usually involves live sessions that allow me to heal the associated traumatic memories through hypnotherapeutic age regression, reprocessing the memories in a safe environment, EFT Therapy, and empowering the client to provide emotional support and protection to their wounded Inner Child. Your Inner Child needs this to counteract the effects of the abuse as well as cognitive restructuring to bridge the gap between your conscious behaviors and their unconscious motivations, so the power to control your life rests firmly in your present and not your past.

For information on in-person sessions with me, visit:

www.asherfoxweightloss.com/personalsessions

If sessions with me personally are geographically difficult, I also provide sessions through Skype.

Negative Core Beliefs: This is almost always attached to basic core beliefs about safety and survival, along with many other negative core beliefs that need to be resolved. Some of the other beliefs include issues around sexuality, the good or bad intentions of others, and self-worth and guilt issues that arose out of the event or events.

Insecurity of the Romantic Partner

You, your weight, and your beliefs about yourself are intimately intertwined with your environment. This is called your personal ecology. When you make significant changes in your life, it effects all other areas of your life, including all of your other relationships. In no area is this effect more pronounced than in romantic relationships.

In my book, *Troublesome Attractions*™, you learn how your negative core beliefs about yourself also influence your selection of a romantic partner. This selection, consciously or unconsciously, directly or indirectly, reinforces your existing core beliefs about yourself.

If you have very low self-esteem, you are more likely to select a partner who also has very low self-esteem who directly or indirectly seeks to make themself feel better by actively or passively working to reinforce your own negative ideas about yourself.

When you begin to change these beliefs and improve your self-esteem, while changing your body, it can have a pronounced effect on the relationship. Romantic partners aren't always happy about these changes because it challenges the fundamental subconscious agreement to preserve both of your existing negative core beliefs upon which your relationship is based.

Over the years, I have dealt with many clients who lost weight, and then found their partners became more insecure. Sometimes this insecurity was based on my client actually receiving more attention from the opposite sex and other times it was completely imagined in their partners' minds. Whether this insecurity was imagined or real, these unhappy partners acted on it in various unpleasant ways that put strain on the relationship and the person who lost weight. While they do not always make the conscious connection as to why, these clients regain weight to avoid dealing with this negative side of their partner and to restore what they perceive as the status quo in their relationship.

Resolving this secondary gain can be complex because it involves much more than just the person's body, but also their romantic relationship and quite frequently the entire family system. In an ideal world, the romantic partner uses this as an opportunity to address their own self-esteem issues and both people grow together into a healthier place. This is covered in much more depth in *Troublesome Attractions*™.

Negative Core Beliefs: The core beliefs surrounding this secondary gain tend to be the same ones that also manifested in the choice of a romantic partner. For example, the core beliefs that "I am unlovable, flawed, and not good enough" and all of the associated low self-esteem that comes from these beliefs, lead to picking a partner with their own self-worth issues who, because of those issues, reacts negatively to their partner's weight loss.

Typically, while the root issue is the same for both partners, it often manifests itself differently. One partner may be passive and overtly self-loathing, while the other partner may appear more confident and attempt to soothe their low self-esteem by dominating the other partner. This dominant partner would likely have chosen someone whose self-esteem was perceived as lower than their own and therefore likely to not leave, thus providing a sense of false security that their insecure self craves.

In our example, the person who is losing weight will experience the fear of losing their partner based on their partner's ever-growing insecurities. Since they believe they are unlovable, they often are unwilling to lose this partner for fear of not being able to find another. They will subconsciously choose to regain weight to avoid this.

With this secondary gain, the relationship itself must be looked at and addressed in one of two ways. In one way, both partners heal. In the other way, the partner who is losing weight and improving their self-esteem reaches the point where they are willing to leave the relationship for someone who is comfortable with the improved version of themselves.

Group Identification

At the heart of this secondary gain is our tribal nature. Quite frequently, food and body size are some of the most powerful ways we connect to others. When it comes to eating, food is often a ritual at the heart of many family get-togethers. When you do not fully indulge, it can lead to family members becoming offended and the non-indulger feels left out and disconnected from the group.

While this dynamic is the most powerful in families, it can also be present in work and social peer groups as well. Overcoming this secondary gain involves resolving any negative core beliefs about your innate self-worth, beliefs around not being included or abandonment, while also learning to savor foods in smaller quantities without overeating.

While less common, sometimes it is not just the eating ritual but also body size that is part of group identification. Usually this takes place within a family system. In these instances, the majority of the people in the group are overweight. When one person starts to lose weight, they experience resentment or experience passive aggressive or ostracizing behavior from the overweight members of the family. Sometimes this is covert, while other times it comes in the overt form of the "you think you're better than us because you lost weight" attitude. Suddenly the person who has lost weight finds themselves not included in the way they were when they were overweight and their size supported the group dynamic.

In these instances, their need to be included and not abandoned often wins out and the person regains their weight to better fit in. This secondary gain is resolved by addressing the same core beliefs that caused them to become overweight. This includes a special emphasis on issues surrounding abandonment and self-worth. It also includes learning appropriate boundaries and healthy assertiveness in determining how you are willing to be treated by others in the group. You also must learn to stand up for yourself through healthy assertiveness when you feel diminished in any way.

Lastly, if you determine that this group is unwilling to support the new and healthier you, it may become necessary for your adult self to make the decision to end or limit your relationship with this group and seek out healthier and more supportive attachments.

Negative Core Beliefs: Common negative core beliefs around this secondary gain deal with issues of abandonment, self-worth, and a lack of healthy boundaries and high self-esteem, usually coupled with attachment-based issues.

Preventing Unfaithfulness

This secondary gain is almost completely unconscious, but I have seen it numerous times, and it can be very powerful. In unsatisfying relationships, it is not uncommon for one or both partners to be tempted to stray from the relationship.

However, when one of these partners has a strong moral objection against cheating, yet finds themselves tempted, excess weight is often a means of preventing themselves from following through. They believe this makes them less attractive and therefore unlikely to be appealing to a potential new lover.

When this secondary gain is present, it's essential to heal the core beliefs keeping them in an unhappy relationship, or steps need to be taken to improve the relationship.

Negative Core Beliefs: Other than the negative core beliefs that keep them in an unsatisfying relationship, the core beliefs that often manifest this secondary gain are not necessarily negative, but are related to your moral center. This is a mechanism to help preserve those moral values, yet all things when taken to the extreme of self-harm, should be reassessed.

Relationship Between Physical Size and Perceived Presence

"Children are meant to be seen and not heard," is a clichéd idea that many parents may not use any longer, but still relay in other ways. I have worked with clients who feel invisible, as if they are just not seen or heard. For some of these clients, the subconsciously held belief that being physically larger makes their presence hard to miss becomes the secondary gain for being overweight.

While this is not the most common secondary gain of weight issues, I have encountered it several times and it is worth looking at. If as a child and throughout your life you felt ignored and unseen, this is a secondary gain worth exploring. You will have an idea that this may apply to you if your negative core beliefs are around those very issues: being ignored, invisible, not noticed, or unheard.

Negative Core Beliefs: This secondary gain is usually attached to the belief that people ignore you, and that you are invisible, not noticed, and unheard. These beliefs are usually part of a more pervasive belief of being unimportant or not good enough.

Avoidance of Sex with Romantic Partner

Frequently, issues with sexual self-esteem and relationship issues with your romantic partner result in either not being fully engaged in physical intimacy or wanting to avoid it altogether. This is a somewhat frequent secondary gain of not losing weight.

The weight serves two purposes. One, it lowers your self-esteem and allows you to give that as an excuse to your romantic partner as to why you do not feel like having sex. Secondly, it is also perceived as diminishing your sexual attractiveness so your partner wants sex less frequently. Addressing core beliefs related to sex, sexual self-esteem, sexual boundaries, romantic partner choice, and the issues within the relationship are key to overcoming this secondary gain.

Negative Core Beliefs: Core beliefs related to this secondary gain revolve around sex and relationship issues. Common beliefs are, "I'm only wanted for sex, and sex is bad." Also, if you have the beliefs of not being good enough or being unlovable and not deserving a happy relationship, withholding sex (either subconsciously or consciously) is a means of sabotaging the relationship and proving your beliefs true.

While this secondary gain is usually linked to the quality of the relationship, sometimes it manifests regardless of the partner involved because of guilt and shame issues around childhood sexual experiences, and core beliefs related to vulnerability and safety that are brought about from physical intimacy or emotional intimacy in a relationship.

Preserving A Habitual Emotional State

Events lead us to form beliefs about ourselves and the world around us in a way that causes us to have emotions that result in symptoms like overeating and being overweight. Not only can these core habits develop around activities and behaviors, but also around ways of thinking and feeling, which creates the boundaries of our emotional comfort zone. Sometimes these feelings are so habitual that the secondary gain can be simply to preserve the state and avoid leaving that emotional comfort zone.

My client Jackson is an example of this.

Due to his unresolved negative core beliefs, Jackson spent most of his life in a state of worry and anxiety. When he didn't have something to worry about, he frantically began searching for something. This really hit home for him when after working for months to have the body he desired, he stepped on the scale for the first time after reaching his goal weight.

He later told me that as soon as he saw the number on the scale and realized he had succeeded, he heard a voice within say, Oh man, what am I going to worry and obsess about now? Jackson realized that in addition to resolving his core beliefs, he needed to change his way of thinking so as not to produce the worry and anxiety he was comfortable with. He needed to develop new neural pathways around peace and joy, not worry and anxiety. He needed a new comfort zone that actually allowed him to be comfortable being happy.

Resolving this secondary gain requires the exact same approach I took with Jackson. After the core beliefs are resolved and the Inner Critic transformed into a healthier voice, the unconscious comfort zone of your prior bad feelings has to be addressed. The first step is of course becoming conscious of your comfort zone while then beginning to incrementally go beyond it. This is accomplished while addressing the emotional reactions that come up through continued use of the techniques you've already learned. You'll find that in different contexts, the Inner Critic can become active again with a whole new list of "shoulds." This is where you will find that the skills you have learned in going from *Fat to Fearless®* can be applied to other areas of your life as well to produce positive transformation.

All of these secondary gains are but a small sample of what I have encountered over the years. Secondary gains are as individual as the people they are attached to.

It can be hard to believe that something you have tried to get rid of your entire life, like your excess weight, is actually providing you with a perceived benefit. In your subconscious mind, this perceived benefit is greater than the pleasure you consciously believe you would get from having the body you want. If you have been trying for years to lose weight only to continue to self-sabotage yourself, there is most likely a subconscious secondary gain that is tied into your negative core beliefs.

From my experience seeing thousands of clients, I can tell you that negative core beliefs are what have been opposing you, but secondary gains almost always develop along with them to avoid dealing with these issues directly and keep such unpleasantness from conscious awareness. Now that you are addressing those negative beliefs and changing them into positive ones that support your long-term weight loss, it is also important to directly uncover and address any secondary gains that are present. In the following exercises you will do exactly that.

EXERCISE: SECONDARY GAIN DETECTIVE

In this exercise, you will go back and review the times in your past you began gaining weight again after losing a significant amount. Let go of any preconceived ideas you have, and think of yourself as a detective, objectively searching the facts and clues to find the hidden secondary gain.

The key to being successful at this exercise is to examine the facts objectively. Imagine being outside of yourself looking in on the situation. Einstein said that a problem can't be solved at the same level at which it was created. Analyzing your past weight loss setbacks and failures from within the subjective state that created them is trying to do exactly that. You must go to another level, the observer's perspective that we talked about previously to do this exercise successfully.

Do these exercises in your *Fat to Fearless*® Success Guide and Workbook or on your own paper.

1. Recall three times you started gaining weight again after losing a significant amount. If there have not been three instances, use however many you can recall.

2. Begin with the first instance and write down the answers to the following questions.

   What changes were there in my life after I lost weight?

   • What changes in my social life?

   • What changes in my career?

   • What changes in my friendships?

   • What changes in my romantic relationships?

   • What changes in my financial life?

   • What changes in lifestyle?

   It is important to log all changes you can think of, even if you do not believe they had anything to do with your weight.

3. Go through each of the changes you found above, and write down the answers to the following questions:

   • How did this change make me feel emotionally? (sad, angry, uncomfortable, etc.)

   • Did this change reinforce any negative core beliefs? (unlovable, not good enough, unsafe, etc.)

4. Now go through each change and ask yourself: "After gaining weight and having things go back to "normal," and even though I did not realize it at the time, did I actually feel more comfortable when they reverted back?" The feeling of comfort we are talking about isn't physical comfort or satisfaction with life, but one of familiarity.

5. From the answers to the above questions, list any secondary gains you may have uncovered even if you don't consciously believe them to be true.

Staying open to these secondary gains, coupled with the work you are already doing, will allow you to better face them. This will lessen their control over you should they arise again. You may find that with the core belief work you are already doing, these secondary gains may never manifest again. Yet being conscious of them, along with the inner transformation you are making and the remaining exercises in this section, will assure they no longer get in your way.

EXERCISE: WHEN I LOSE WEIGHT I WILL . . .

Now that you've reviewed your past weight loss ups and downs from an objective standpoint searching for secondary gains, use your future plans in much the same way that you did your past.

1. Make a list of all the things you tell yourself you're going to do when you lose weight. For the most part, these should be things you feel your weight is currently holding you back from doing.

These may be things like:

A. I will date more.

B. I will be more social.

C. I will take more of a leadership role at work.

D. I will take some really great photos and put them on social media.

E. I will go back to school.

F. I will come out of my "shell."

2. Now take each of these items and plug them into the following sentence. You've done stem sentences several times, and you know the importance of answering from your first gut instinct without censoring the answer intellectually with your conscious mind.

Complete this sentence:

I don't ___(insert goal/activity)___ **now** because I am afraid that_____.

Your first response may have been your weight. But I want you to go beyond that as an answer. Below is an example:

First Response: I don't begin dating more now because I'm afraid women/men *will think I'm fat.*

Second Response (not answering with weight): I don't begin dating more now because I'm afraid women/men *will not be attracted to me.*

Complete this exercise for each of the goal activities on your list.

3. Now analyze each of your non-weight related answers. Consider the possibility that your weight isn't why you fear doing the activity, but instead your weight protects you from finding out that what you fear isn't based on your body but inherent to you as a person.

In our example, the core fear (core belief) is that you are unattractive or ugly. As long as you are overweight, you are able to hold on to the possibility that this isn't true and not risk finding out that it is. You can believe that you are attractive and the reason you perceive the world doesn't see it is your weight. This, in our example, is the secondary gain to the weight. The fear of losing weight and finding out you might not be attractive anyway is greater than the conscious desire to lose weight. From this example, you can easily see how secondary gains develop to avoid dealing with the underlying issue, which is typically the negative core belief that needs to be resolved.

4. Now, in your *Fat to Fearless*® Success Guide and Workbook, fill in the appropriate blanks with which of your above answers may be potential secondary gains to maintaining excess weight.

After completing this exercise you should have a list of potential secondary gains to add to your list from the first exercise in the section. In the next chapter, you will begin eliminating your secondary gains on the last step of your *Fat to Fearless*® journey.

SUMMARY

Key Points

- "Secondary gains" is the psychological term for unconscious motivations we have for maintaining behaviors or conditions that we consciously want to change.

- Almost everyone who suffers from lifelong weight issues has secondary gains that are part of why they've never been successful at losing weight.

- Secondary gains develop as a maladaptive means to keep us from directly dealing with issues we want to deny and avoid. Because of this, we are often in collusion with our subconscious in keeping secondary gains hidden. These keep us from having to confront issues in our lives we would rather ignore.

- Being willing to confront the true issue behind the hidden benefits of being overweight (avoiding intimacy for instance) is necessary to dismantling your secondary gains, which is necessary for permanent weight loss.

- One of the keys to uncovering secondary gains is being able to objectively look at the circumstances surrounding all areas of your life during periods of time that you've gained and lost weight.

- Psychologist Carl Jung said all neurosis is an attempt to avoid legitimate suffering. This means that a habit like using food to deal with emotional pain is a way of avoiding dealing with the true underlying issue.

- By dealing directly with the issue underlying the secondary gain, you eliminate the need for the secondary gain. In other words, if whatever being overweight is designed to keep you from doing you do anyway, your subconscious no longer has a reason to keep you overweight because it's not serving the subconscious purpose it was designed to serve. This is of course assuming you've also, through your previous *Fat to Fearless®* work, resolved the negative core beliefs associated with these issues.

What This Has To Do With Weight Loss

If you have managed to go through school, hold a job, raise a family, or accomplish any significant goal in your life that required overcoming difficulty and exerting willpower, then why have you never been able to achieve long-term weight loss? This is an even more powerful question when most people say that reaching their weight loss goals is more important than most other difficult goals they've reached.

The answer lies in understanding secondary gains, which are the hidden motivations you have for sabotaging your weight loss efforts. With other difficult goals you've achieved, your conscious and subconscious minds were aligned to mobilize enough of your resources to overcome the obstacles that stood in your path, resist temptation, and persevere until you achieved what you set out to do.

With weight loss, especially if being overweight has been a life-long struggle, it is common that a part of you is actually working against you and not only prevents you from using all of your internal resources to stay motivated and on track to lose weight, but actually turns some of your own resources against you. Achieving permanent weight loss requires uncovering these hidden motivations, taking them from unconscious to conscious, and looking at them under the light of truth. When you understand why you have been holding yourself back, apply your adult reasoning mind to these "reasons" while using the *Fat to Fearless®* methodology to diffuse the emotional components of the block, you are able to align your conscious and subconscious minds towards achieving your long-term weight loss goals in much the same way you have overcome life's other challenges.

You Are Ready To Move To The Next Chapter When

- You understand the concept of secondary gains and how they may be the source of your weight loss self-sabotage.

- You have watched the tutorial video for this chapter (if you have the full *Fat to Fearless*® program).

- You have completed the exercises for this chapter in the Success Guide and Workbook (if you have the full *Fat to Fearless*® program).

CHAPTER 24

LIVING FEARLESSLY

The final step on your *Fat to Fearless*® journey is very much entwined with what you just learned about secondary gains. Secondary gains are the unconscious motivations you have for staying overweight that are designed to protect you from having to confront your real underlying issues and negative core beliefs.

Secondary gains are by definition a neurosis. While there are many variations of the definition of a neurosis, in terms of secondary gains it is defined as a psychological state often characterized by anxiety, avoidance behavior, and unconscious defense mechanisms often triggered by unresolved conflicts. Neuroses have no biological or neurological component, and the maladaptive behaviors, such as overeating and being overweight, are not so far outside of the social norm as to prohibit societal functioning.

To put it more simply: When being overweight is a secondary gain, it is a neurosis in that it is a maladaptive behavior to avoid dealing with the true subconscious/conscious conflict between what you believe you consciously want, your negative core beliefs, and your subconscious/conscious fears that the negative core beliefs may be true.

Carl Jung, the founder of analytical psychology, said that "neurosis is always a substitute for legitimate suffering." (The passage comes from his 1938 *Psychology and Religion*.) What this means is that most would rather stay unconscious of their internal conflicts, dealing with whatever neurotic symptoms (such as emotional or binge eating) have manifested as a result of not dealing with the real issue, rather than suffer the associated pain of bringing these conflicts to consciousness and resolving them.

These subconscious motivations to stay overweight are often the most difficult obstacles to overcome to permanently losing your weight. You could have successfully done all of the work in the program up to this point, but you may still fail to lose weight and keep it off if you don't dismantle your secondary gains. The positive part is that eliminating the secondary gains by using the methods you're going to learn now often results in the most dramatic progress toward weight loss than you've experienced during any other part of the program.

As usual, the problem begins with our negative core beliefs. These core beliefs make us feel as if we are "not good enough" or deficient in some way. However, while we may be unaware of our negative subconscious core beliefs, or at the very least not fully aware of how much they influence us, our conscious mind continues to hope and dream.

We develop goals and things we want to accomplish that are often in direct opposition to what we truly believe about our capabilities and ourselves at the deepest level. This conflict between our subconscious and our conscious is the root of almost all of our repeated failures to accomplish the things in life that we consciously believe are so very important to us. You've also learned that our subconscious takes our beliefs as instructions for what is true and sets out to construct our lives based on that "truth." Being overweight and repeatedly failing to lose it is one of the ways our subconscious proves to ourselves we aren't good enough and are flawed (if those are part of our negative subconscious belief system).

To make matters worse, we develop a fear—of which sometimes we are aware and other times we aren't—around the conflict between what we say we want to do and what we truly believe we can do. Typically, this fear is a pre-conscious fear, which means that it is not being repressed into the subconscious, yet not readily accessible in our conscious mind either. It hovers somewhere in between, like that word or name on the tip of your tongue. This fear is some variation of: *What if my negative core beliefs are true, and I'm really not good enough, smart enough, etc. regardless of my weight.* To understand the significance of this, it's important to understand the degree to which most people consciously deny their negative core beliefs.

In the beginning of this book, I said that many people are aware (to some degree) of their negative core beliefs, yet many are unaware and often in complete denial. I've worked with hundreds of clients whose lives were in complete shambles because of decisions they made that reflected a complete lack of self-respect and self-love. They still refused to accept that they had any beliefs that they weren't good enough or deficient in any way, despite what the evidence of their lives indicated. No matter how many times I tried to make them understand that someone who truly loves themself and has the core beliefs that they are worthwhile and valuable does not engage in self-sabotaging decision making, they refused to acknowledge it at all.

When people don't want to face their fears that their negative core beliefs may be true, they put subconscious obstacles in place to protect them from consciously having to deal with the issue. These obstacles are secondary gains, in that the obstacle has a hidden benefit of protecting them from the fear involved in confronting their limiting core beliefs. Quite often being overweight is the obstacle that is chosen to avoid facing this internal conflict.

It typically goes like this:

Negative Core Beliefs Develop (Events → Beliefs → Emotions → Symptoms → Reinforce Core Beliefs)

Once you have these negative core beliefs, they subsequently create emotions and symptoms. If you're reading this book, emotional eating and being overweight are probably at least some of the symptoms that developed.

You consciously develop goals that are in conflict with these limiting core beliefs. You consciously tell yourself you have what it takes to reach these goals and will do it as soon as you lose your weight.

In spite of consciously believing you will be able to accomplish these goals as soon as you lose weight, a pre-conscious fear develops that your core beliefs may be true and you may not have what it takes to reach these goals even if you lose the weight and have the body you want.

The fear of finding out that you may not be able to reach your goals because you don't *"have what it takes, aren't good enough, etc."* grows until you put an obstacle in your path that keeps you from having to face this fear of not being good enough. Since you have already told yourself that you won't try to do whatever the goal is until after you lose weight, not being able to lose weight becomes the perfect obstacle. At this point, being overweight serves two functions: it *subconsciously* proves to you that your negative core beliefs are true (not good enough, ugly, etc.) while *consciously* allowing you to preserve hope that you are good enough, etc. and will achieve your goals just as soon as you lose weight. As long as you never lose the weight, you never have to risk failure and finding out you really *"aren't good enough, are unlovable, etc."* This subconscious fear is ultimately greater than your conscious desire to lose weight, resulting in constant weight loss self-sabotage every time you come close to reaching your weight loss goals and eliminating your self-imposed obstacle to doing the things you have been avoiding "because" of your weight.

Let's break it down further:

1. Through the subconscious mechanisms you've learned about, you develop the negative core beliefs that you aren't good enough and are unlovable (for example).

2. Unpleasant emotions (fear, sadness, anger, for example) develop because of these beliefs. You turn to food to self-soothe, which makes you overweight, which in turn causes you to feel even more strongly that you aren't good enough and are unlovable.

3. Despite all of this going on subconsciously, consciously you develop goals for yourself that are in conflict with your negative core beliefs. In our example, let's say that the goal is to find a mate that will completely love you and accept you for yourself.

4. Consciously, you believe you are lovable and deserve this, but your subconscious core beliefs tell you something different.

5. Because to function effectively in life you must have some hope that your dreams will come true, you must find a way of preserving this hope at all costs. When you begin to develop fears that your subconscious beliefs about being flawed, not good enough, a loser, ugly, etc., may be true (which would take away your hope), an unwillingness to uncover and face this fear causes you to subconsciously put a "prerequisite" that must be met before you attempt to reach your goals. This prerequisite is almost always a symptom that developed from the same negative core beliefs that you are avoiding dealing with. For emotional eaters and weight loss self-sabotagers, losing weight is usually the prerequisite.

6. In our example, you would set up weight loss as a prerequisite for dating and searching for this mate. Therefore, as long as you stay overweight you are able to continue to tell yourself you deserve to find a mate and are worthy of love and it will happen as soon as you reach your goal weight. If you lose the weight, however, you may actually have to confront the true fear that you are fundamentally

not good enough and unlovable, regardless of what your body size or shape.

7. Therefore, every time you get close to losing your weight and eliminating your self-imposed barrier to dating, you are also getting closer to potentially finding out that you really are unlovable and not good enough. The fear of facing this causes you to subconsciously regain your weight or never reach your final weight loss goal.

This is the root of how weight loss as a secondary gain often develops as a coping mechanism to keep us from facing our core fears about ourselves and finding out they're true. If you have goals, hopes, and dreams you want to accomplish that are in conflict with your subconscious beliefs about your worth and capabilities, as well as a conscious or subconscious fear about finding out that those negative thoughts about yourself might be true, then you subconsciously create an obstacle for yourself that keeps you from facing that fear. This obstacle is a secondary gain, and if you are reading this book, the obstacle you've most likely set up for yourself is body fat.

The symptom of being overweight is often a way of not only subconsciously proving that your negative core beliefs are accurate, but also protecting you from consciously confirming that accuracy. By avoiding facing your fear you can continue to function with, and be motivated by, hope and your plans for the future. This is the secondary gain of being overweight. It creates a "perfect" balanced system of keeping you safe by avoiding you ever going beyond the subconscious comfort zone defined by your negative core beliefs, while also creating motivation to continue to strive. Your subconscious and conscious minds conspire to create both the carrot and the stick to keep you "safe" and functional exactly where you are.

The secondary gain functions to:

1. Subconsciously prove your core beliefs are true.

2. Protect you from dealing with the pain of confronting the core belief and finding they are true (they're not by the way).

3. Preserve conscious hope (important for functioning).

4. Act as a synergistic system that keeps you functioning with hope while also making sure you never go beyond the established guidelines of your negative core beliefs.

My client Ingrid illustrates the concept:

Ingrid had always dreamed of being a model, yet she believed her weight stood in her way. She wasn't extremely overweight, but definitely didn't have the body that she saw in magazines. When I began seeing Ingrid as a client, she told me that she knew she had the face, skills, and attitude to be a successful model, and the extra 30 pounds she carried was all that stood in her way. Because she believed being a model was so important to her, she couldn't understand why every time she got close to reaching her goal weight she would compulsively start eating bad foods, lose her motivation to exercise, and within a few short months be back where she started.

Using many of the techniques you've learned in this program, we uncovered her core beliefs. Because she was in such conscious denial about these beliefs, I used the Fat to Fearless® hypnotherapeutic age regression protocols in a live session to go back to events in her childhood where the beliefs were formed. When we were done, it was clear she had the following core beliefs: I'm second best, I'm not attractive, I'm unlovable.

Through our sessions together, Ingrid learned that her weight, along with self-sabotaging many of her romantic relationships, was a result of her subconscious working to prove these beliefs to be true. During a particularly emotional breakdown, she admitted that now that she was getting more in touch with her emotions and becoming more willing to face what she'd always suspected that she believed about herself at the deepest level, she was also aware she had a fear that maybe she wasn't as pretty as she thought she was. She feared that even if she lost the weight her modeling dreams were hopeless.

This was when I helped Ingrid see how her weight issues were not only designed to subconsciously prove her negative beliefs about herself to be true, but they protected her from consciously facing the fear of confronting those beliefs. Every time she got close to reaching her goal weight, she also got closer to potentially finding out she wasn't pretty enough to be a model regardless of her weight and subsequently losing her dream. As long as she was overweight, she could tell herself she was attractive enough to reach her modeling goals, and it was going to happen as soon as she shed those excess pounds.

At this point, the work with Ingrid became about her accepting that not facing this fear and dealing with these negative core beliefs would cause a lifetime of suffering far greater than whatever the outcome of her modeling aspirations. The choice was simply to spend a lifetime hoping to achieve something her subconscious would never let her do out of fear of failure or overcome that fear, resolve the negative beliefs, and move forward with a life constructed out of more positive beliefs.

Ultimately, after working together to resolve her negative core beliefs and her secondary gains around weight, which were to protect her from confirming her fear that she was unattractive, she was able to lose the weight. At this point, it was time for her to find out if she really had a shot of being a model.

But what if our negative core beliefs *are* true!

This is where some of the real magic of this process happens. After resolving her negative core beliefs and the secondary gains around being overweight, she was easily able to shed her remaining pounds and realized that her desire to be a model was a reaction to her fear that she was not attractive. It was a subconsciously driven manifestation of her desire to receive conscious external validation. In other words, if she was accepted as a model it was objective proof that she wasn't unattractive.

Once she changed her core beliefs to believe that she was beautiful, regardless of whether or not she was perfect (one of the things we had to dismantle was the Inner Critic Cognitive Distortion of all-or-nothing thinking), the driving force behind her desire to model disappeared, and she became interested in other things. It wasn't that she wasn't pretty enough to model; she just didn't *need* to do it anymore to prove to herself that she was beautiful. She found true beauty within.

This brings us to another very important principle: After resolving your negative core beliefs, your value comes from within instead of from outside yourself based on your accomplishments or the opinions of others. Subsequently, the things those old negative beliefs held you back from become irrelevant to your self-esteem and no longer an indicator of your value and worth.

In Ingrid's example, you can see how the secondary gain, the hidden unconscious motivation, to maintaining her weight was avoiding the possible pain of finding out she was unattractive regardless of her excess pounds. Her weight not only served to confirm subconsciously her negative core beliefs but allowed her to consciously maintain hope for the future in spite of those beliefs. By confronting her fears and resolving them *before* reaching her goal weight, she eliminated her last subconscious block to losing weight by making the prerequisite of weight loss an ineffective obstacle for avoiding dealing with the issue (thus eliminating it as a secondary gain) and actually validated her hope through the process of being fearless.

Here is another example from my own life.

I had always wanted to take my work to the international level and consciously believed that I had all the skills and abilities to do that. The more success I had with clients, the greater my desire to offer my programs to a larger audience and help more people. I had done some work in film and radio early in my career, and the feedback I received made me believe even more in my abilities to translate my work into media for a larger audience. My challenge was that even though I had eliminated my excess weight, and most would even consider me fit (using the same Fat to Fearless® process you've gone through), I still felt I didn't look good enough for how I wanted to present myself in this larger arena.

Even though most of my clients were obese when they began and were thrilled to have lost their excess weight and were happy with their healthier and slimmer selves, the standard I set for myself was much higher. I'm sure my early years in the fitness industry played a significant role in my belief that before stepping out onto an international stage I needed to obtain that fitness model body. It seemed the harder I tried, the more that body eluded me.

As time went by and news of my success with one-on-one clients and group sessions grew, my circle of influence and those that knew of my work grew as well. I began receiving more offers to work on a larger scale. I was approached with offers of radio shows, local TV appearances, and an international seminar. Eventually these opportunities became too good to continue passing up and despite feeling uncomfortable and not ready because I didn't have the perfect physique I wanted, I reached a point where I accepted that these opportunities were presented to me for a reason. I chose to move forward.

I began writing this book, prepared to launch my own radio show, and developed partnerships with industry leaders around the world. I did this to reach my long-term goal of taking my work to an international level and increasing the number of people who I could help through my programs. While I was uncomfortable going through photo shoots and videos, not having the complete fitness physique I wanted, I was able to move through my discomfort because I consciously knew it wasn't necessary for the type of work I was doing. It was only something I personally wanted because of psychological programming from my years in the fitness industry.

As a matter of fact, many of the consultants I worked with advised me against having that type of stereotypical physique, believing it would be a turn-off to my more overweight clients and would have made me less approachable and relatable. In addition, my before and after photos were already so extreme from how I looked now as opposed to when I weighed 300 pounds, it would almost make my transformation seem unbelievable if I were any more "in shape." I moved forward toward my goals with my current body in spite of my desire for the physique that had eluded me in the prior months. A strange thing then happened the closer I got to my international launch.

While I consciously believed I had what it took to work at this new level, doubt began to seep in. I was surprised because had you asked me six months earlier, I not only would've told you that I had what it took, but also that I felt as if it was what I was "made fore" and that I knew I was meant to help people on a larger scale. Yet, the closer my dreams came to fruition, the more my doubts grew. My Inner Critic, for the first time in a long time, became very active again telling me things like, "Who do you think you are to do this?" and "You probably don't have the right type of image to translate your work into this type of media." I was actually surprised when this began because by going through all of the processes I've guided you through so far, I thought I had resolved these negative beliefs.

This leads us to the following important principle: You don't fully know if you have resolved your negative core beliefs until you're actively doing what you allowed these limiting beliefs to hold you back from doing.

While I had always known my weight issues were a manifestation of my negative core beliefs and the emotional eating that resulted from them, what I hadn't realized was that being overweight had been a secondary gain to keep me from facing the fear I wasn't good enough to make my larger dreams come true. Because I hadn't consciously realized this was the case, I had only resolved my subconscious roadblocks to the degree that had allowed me to lose my excess weight, not to the degree that had allowed me to move forward doing the things I had always said I would do once I reached my weight loss goal.

Put simply, I had resolved my negative core beliefs enough to believe I was good enough, lovable enough, and worthy of being slim and not overweight, but not necessarily worthy of reaching my bigger dreams. As a matter of fact, what was left of those negative core beliefs had resulted in me setting the bar higher so that it wasn't enough to be slim and healthy to begin moving toward my big goals—I needed the perfect physique too.

You may be thinking, "So what? If I resolved my issues enough to lose weight that would be enough for me!" But that is a very precarious position to be in. Remember, our goal is to lose weight and keep it off for a lifetime. To not fully resolve your negative core beliefs is like treating an infection only until the symptoms subside and not eliminating it completely. Eventually, when your immune system is low enough, the infection may find its way back. For you, the equivalent of a low immune system would be extreme times of stress or change that might cause your negative core beliefs and the subsequent negative emotions to flare up to the point where you again reach for food. This is why it's important to do the work completely.

For example, once my own fears and insecurities began to show themselves as I came closer to achieving my dreams, the more I found my old urges to eat mindlessly returning. I was subconsciously trying to use my weight to again put a barrier in front of me to avoid facing the possibility of failure. Fortunately, using the tools that I've taught you in this book, I was able to use this experience as a tool to fully dismantle what was left of those old negative core beliefs.

I was able to do this through the following three important steps.

1. I identified that the way I felt about my body was keeping me from pursuing something I wanted and accepted the possibility that my fear of failure might be causing me to use my remaining body image issues as a secondary gain.

2. I made a conscious choice to move forward with doing it anyway in spite of not having reached my complete body-related goals.

3. As I moved forward, in spite of not having the perfect physique, I resolved what was left of the negative core beliefs holding me back, by working through the discomfort using the *Fat to Fearless*® system. By doing this, I made my body issues ineffective as a secondary gain, eliminating the subconscious reason for keeping me from getting the physique I wanted.

When I say the secondary gain is ineffective, I mean that it's no longer doing its job of protecting you from failure by keeping you from taking action, and therefore the secondary gain typically falls apart. When whatever challenge you've put in place to keep you from facing your fear becomes ineffective because you are moving forward in spite of it, the subconscious no longer has a reason for actively keeping you from overcoming that challenge. In my case, once I moved forward despite not having the perfect body I wanted, I was able to easily begin making progress toward that goal again without my subconscious working against me.

Let me explain more simply. Remember, the secondary gain is designed to protect you from facing the fear of failure that comes from whatever you tell yourself you're going to do when you lose weight. Specifically, the fear is that even when you're no longer overweight, you still won't be able to do the things you want to do. For this reason, even if you've done all of the other work in the program, your subconscious is going to resist you losing weight because it is the last line of defense to keep you from facing these fears and possibly the disappointment that may come.

When you begin facing these fears anyway, even when you haven't reached your goal weight, the subconscious no longer has a reason to use excess body fat as a way to hold you back from facing your fears because that body fat is no longer holding you back. It ceases to be an effective secondary gain. Once this final secondary gain to being overweight is eliminated, you no longer have subconscious resistance holding you back from reaching your body goals.

Before we begin applying this to you so you can take your final step on the *Fat to Fearless*® journey, let me give you one more example.

Laura came to me about two issues that were far more entwined than she realized. She needed help to lose weight and find a long-term relationship. After going through the *Fat to Fearless*® program we identified the negative core beliefs that led to the emotions that she was soothing through food. We also balanced her pain/pleasure scale on a daily basis so that she wasn't turning to food to compensate. And through the use of hypnotherapy audios, we used emotion and repetition to reprogram many of her habits to achieve healthy weight loss. All that was left was to dismantle the secondary gains around her weight.

One of her negative core beliefs we specifically worked on was that relationships mean a loss of control. It was in working on this that we uncovered that, since she didn't want to date until she reached her goal weight, the secondary gain to being overweight was protecting her from "losing control" by getting in a relationship.

Because of the work we had already done together to disempower her Inner Critic, heal and strengthen her Inner Child, and transform her negative core beliefs, with my support she decided to begin dating before reaching her goal weight, even though this was uncomfortable for her.

In the beginning, all of her fears and doubts surfaced. However, after making it through the first few dates, her Inner Critic quieted, she journaled with her Inner Child any time her emotional self needed reinforcing, and used her Hypnotherapy Audio Sessions to harness the power of repetition and emotion to program her subconscious mind to support her.

After she rescheduled a couple of sessions and I hadn't heard from her in a few weeks, I emailed to check on her progress. She apologized for not being in touch. She was having so much fun dating that between her work schedule and after-hour activities she hadn't had much time. She even believed that she had met someone that was going to turn out to be a long-term boyfriend. Since her relationship issues were resolving, I also asked her about the other subject we worked on together—her remaining weight loss. She said, "You know, it's the strangest thing. Since I've been dating and enjoying myself, I haven't really thought much about my weight in the obsessive way I did before. What's the most strange is that I broke my weight loss plateau and lost an extra five pounds in the past two weeks. I guess you were right, I was using my weight to keep me from dating, and once I started dating anyway, I had no reason to keep the weight on since it wasn't holding me back anyway."

The last I spoke with Laura a few months ago, she had reached her final goal weight, and even though the guy she was seeing previously didn't turn out to be a long-term relationship, she was still actively dating and enjoying the process of looking for that person.

It's time to begin applying these principles to yourself. In the next four steps, you'll begin living life fearlessly and resolve what may be left of your former negative core beliefs.

Step 1: Feel the Fear and Do It Anyway

The first step in living a fearless life is realizing that while there may always be fear of some type, like all seemingly negative emotions, it doesn't have to hold us back. Fear is designed to let us know when something is unsafe, to keep us from doing something that may bring us harm. The challenge comes when we misinterpret and mislabel as unsafe those things beyond our emotional comfort zone. When those things can actually improve our lives, and fear subsequently holds us back, it is to our detriment.

Through the *Fat to Fearless*® process, you have learned to redefine your personal boundaries as you change the negative core beliefs that previously defined them. Yet, realizing your previous boundaries don't need to define you and that you are capable of doing and being so much more (losing weight and keeping it off being only a beginning), doesn't mean you're actually going to cross those boundaries or realize that potential. That's because the ability to act doesn't necessarily mean that we do. That's why the first step to live fearlessly is to take action in spite of any remaining fear.

This is where your conscious adult self must be strong enough to make the decision to move forward, or accept that you are allowing fear and discomfort to hold you back.

If you remember, the first steps I took on my journey to finally resolve my negative core beliefs and living fearlessly was that I was able to identify that the way I felt about my body kept me from pursuing what I wanted, and I chose to move forward with doing it anyway.

Just like me, the first step for you is to actually begin living life by doing those things you tell yourself you can't do unless you reach your final weight loss goal. Until you actually do what you held yourself back from, you may never reach your final weight loss goal because your weight may serve as a secondary gain to protect you from fear of failure.

My former client Frederick is a good example.

Frederick always wanted to be more dynamic, more front and center at work. He knew that leading presentations during meetings was the quickest way in his work environment to get noticed by his supervisors and be fast-tracked for promotions. Yet, he always shied away from the opportunity to do this because of how uncomfortable being overweight made him feel in front of groups. He always believed that if he stood up in front of a group of colleagues, obviously not being able to control his own eating, how could they take him seriously and put him in charge of anything else.

Frederick and I worked together, and he quickly stopped his emotional eating while becoming more assertive and confident. Once Frederick felt comfortable with continuing on his own, he stopped his sessions with the plan of calling me if he had any difficulties and we needed to reinforce the work we had done. When he stopped seeing me, he had already lost 50 pounds and still had 100 pounds left to lose.

Frederick called me about a year later because no matter what he did, he couldn't lose the last 20 pounds. What Frederick hadn't realized consciously that I quickly picked up from our renewed sessions was that he told himself that when he reached his goal weight he would actively begin moving his career forward by beginning to do those work presentations he'd avoided for so long. I helped Frederick uncover that the hidden and unconscious motivation for not losing that last 20 pounds was to avoid leading those work presentations and possibly failing.

On one hand, Frederick consciously believed he would do great in these presentations, yet deep down—once he looked at it more closely—he did have some fear around it. He didn't have to look at this fear before because it really didn't matter— he was 100 pounds away from having to face the possibility that maybe he didn't have what it took to lead those presentations and get promoted. Now that all but 20 pounds of his excess weight was gone, he was in striking distance of either the success he always consciously believed he could achieve or the failure that he subconsciously feared was true.

At this point, Frederick had to make a decision. Did he follow the Fat to Fearless® protocol and live fearlessly without attaching an arbitrary weight goal that needed to be met first, or did he let his fears attached to the belief that he needed to lose that 20 pounds first hold him back.

Frederick chose to follow the Fat to Fearless® protocol, and in spite of being 20 pounds from his goal weight, he took advantage of the next opportunity to lead a project and to do a presentation.

While it wasn't easy for Frederick, because it brought up all of the remaining fragments of the negative core beliefs he'd been working to resolve, he used what he had learned in the *Fat to Fearless*® program and worked through that discomfort and moved forward. We'll see how Frederick did that as we follow him through the remaining steps, but for now it's time for you to do Step One yourself.

Turn to the appropriate section in your Success Guide and Workbook and do the following exercise.

EXERCISE: FEEL THE FEAR AND DO IT ANYWAY!

1. Review the list you made in the prior exercise, those things you were holding yourself back from doing because of your weight, and select one to begin doing now before you've reached your final goal. You might choose to begin with a smaller goal and work your way up to larger ones.

2. Before turning the page in this book (that means right now!), take one solid step to move toward doing this sooner rather than later. In Frederick's case, he checked the intranet at his work to see what upcoming projects needed someone to volunteer to lead. For you, it may be researching the best dating website in your area, looking up dance schools, or ordering college catalogs. Whatever it is, do it now because you want positive momentum on your side. Fear grows in the space filled with unfocused inaction.

3. Now make a time commitment to begin this activity you felt you couldn't do until you lost weight. For Frederick, he emailed his boss letting him know he wanted to take the lead on the project beginning the next month. For you this may look something like:

    • Deciding to put yourself on an Internet dating site within the next week and begin dating ASAP.

- Signing up to audition for a play at a local theater you were too self-conscious to do because you first felt you needed to reach your goal weight.

- Calling your friends and becoming more social again; perhaps going dancing again, even if you're unable to fit into your old skinny jeans.

Make a solid scheduling commitment right now. If you can't actually determine a time right now because of possibly needing more information or conferring with someone else, schedule a time to take that next step in getting that information and continue moving yourself forward through whatever steps are necessary until you have a definite time commitment to begin.

The one prerequisite for this step is that you are not to schedule it based on anything having to do with your weight. In other words, if you could do it this week but you schedule it three weeks from now because you believe you will have lost a few more pounds, then it defeats the purpose. You've essentially told yourself that you won't do this thing you fear as long as you don't lose the weight, which makes not losing the weight a secondary gain and ensures you sabotage your weight loss to avoid following through on the thing you fear.

Once you've decided on what this activity is and have taken the necessary steps to schedule it, move on to Step 2 of the protocol.

Step 2: Working Through Fear

From my own story, you may remember what my next step was to conquer secondary gains and defeat what remained of my negative core beliefs. I moved forward in spite of the obstacle I had placed in front of myself to protect me from possible failure *because I had done enough work on myself that I was able to work through the discomfort.*

This is why in the beginning of this section I talked about the importance of not moving forward until you have adequately gone through all the preceding sections and done the work involved.

It's important to actively apply everything you've learned up to this point and deal with the remaining doubts and fears as they come up. While it may be uncomfortable, when you're able to defeat what your Inner Critic says about your abilities (while empowering your Inner Child and ensuring you're getting enough healthy pleasure to offset the discomfort), you will find this easier to do than you may realize.

Let's return to Frederick.

At first Frederick was excited to have taken the step forward he had wanted to take for a long time. However, as he began doing the work and the date of the presentation came closer, the remnants of those old negative core beliefs became active. His Inner Critic told him things like, "Nobody's going to take you seriously. Up until now they at least think you're good at what you do because they haven't seen your flaws; now you're putting your shortcomings on display! Maybe it's not too late to get out of this."

Because of his Inner Critic's renewed attacks, he began to doubt himself even more and feared he wasn't good enough (as you've learned, these are the Inner Child's fears and emotions being triggered as a result of the Inner Critic's negative self-attacks). He began to feel the urge to eat again, which would:

- Soothe his negative emotions.

- Cause him to gain weight, which would again reaffirm his former negative core beliefs.

- Re-empower his weight as a secondary gain to hold him back from moving forward with the presentation and protect him from failure.

This is where Step 2 comes in. By doing the things you told yourself you couldn't do because of your weight, you bring up the last bit of these negative core beliefs so you can have the opportunity to apply everything you've learned to finish them off in the context of living a fearless life.

Fred immediately:

- Looked for cognitive distortions in what his Inner Critic was telling him, applied challenge questions to them and saw how quickly they unraveled in light of the truth.

- He made the Inner Critics voice humorous sounding, while adjusting its volume to get quieter the more that it spoke (adjusted submodalities) and did this until it became a habit.

- He used his Inner Child Journal to talk with his emotional self about the fears coming up and assured his Inner Child he was more than capable of the task at hand.

- Anytime he doubted himself, he turned to his Evidence Journal to provide proof he had all of the qualities needed to be successful.

- He created a mental movie trailer filled with positive emotion that showed him successfully and confidently delivering his presentation and winning the respect and admiration of his peers and supervisors. He played it at least once in his mind every day leading up to the event.

- He created a separate set of affirmations from his first set that were specific to his ability to successfully do this presentation and get the outcome he desired.

- Because he realized he would be going outside of his comfort zone, which essentially meant adding pain, he made sure he scheduled extra pleasurable activities that weren't food related to make sure he didn't go back to old eating habits to compensate for a pleasure deficit.

- He found positive memories in which he felt confident and courageous and used them to create anchors for himself that he used every time he practiced his presentation, and also used during his actual presentation.

He actively listened to his "Feel the Fear and Do It Anyway" Hypnotherapy Session included in his *Fat to Fearless*® Hypnotherapy Audios.

Fred learned that living a fearless life is about feeling the fear, doing it anyway, and using whatever uncomfortable emotions that come up as an opportunity to apply his *Fat to Fearless*® skills to further resolve whatever was left of his former negative beliefs. Now it's time for you to do the same.

In the corresponding section of your Success Guide and Workbook, make a list of all the skills you've acquired in going through the *Fat to Fearless*® process. Use everything you've learned to constantly overcome any emotional fears, doubts, or blocks that keep you from moving forward fearlessly. Specifically, I suggest that at the very least you:

1. Make a mental movie trailer filled with positive emotions of you successfully doing this activity.

2. Create positive emotional anchors to use while practicing or doing this activity that can be applied to help you overcome any emotional obstacles that present themselves during the process.

3. Create a custom set of affirmations that continue to reinforce your new positive core beliefs while adding specific affirmations related to you successfully doing this activity.

4. Listen to your "Feel the Fear and Do It Anyway" Hypnotherapy Session every day between when you make the commitment to live fearlessly (Now!) and the date you've set to follow through on that commitment.

If you feel emotional discomfort, move forward anyway, and use the fear to further empower yourself as you dismantle the secondary gain. The next step explains further.

Step 3: Make The Secondary Gain Ineffective

Now that you are actively doing the activity you told yourself you couldn't do until you reached your goal weight, you have completely diffused your weight as a secondary gain. Remember your weight was a secondary gain because it protected you from facing the fear that your negative core beliefs might be true, and you were incapable of living the life you wanted even if you lost weight. By facing these fears directly in spite of your weight, you eliminate excess fat as a useful tool for your subconscious to use to protect you from failure because you're doing it anyway.

Once extra body fat is no longer an effective tool to hold you back, you eliminate the need to subconsciously self-sabotage your weight loss, and you notice it is even easier to move forward with reaching any remaining healthy weight loss goals you have.

To further reinforce the irrelevance of your weight to achieving your dreams, do the following exercise.

1. Create a new Evidence Journal as you go through the process of living life fearlessly. Collect evidence that specifically shows your weight really wasn't an obstacle to these activities, since you're doing them now. In Fred's journal, he kept record of all of the positive feedback he'd gotten from his presentation as well as how great he felt for having done it. Anytime in the future that he started to let the remaining pounds he was in the process of losing hold him back, he referred to the Evidence Journal to show him proof that he didn't need to.

2. Write a letter of resignation from your "excess weight" to your subconscious. In this letter, you will "speak" as if you are your excess weight, and you will resign from the job of holding yourself back and limiting your experience of life. This letter can be a powerful symbol for you to review along with your Evidence Journal.

Step 4: Begin Again

Now that you successfully have done or are doing one of the things you used to let weight hold you back from doing, you have a powerfully positive experience to allow you to fearlessly do the next thing on your list. With each new activity you do that reinforces your value and your ability to live life fearlessly regardless of how much you weigh, it will be easier to continue losing weight. Also, the weight loss process is no longer a joyless one where you deny yourself all that you deserve until some magic number on the scale says you're worthwhile. Instead, it is a process where you lose weight while celebrating your self-worth.

EXERCISE: BEGIN AGAIN

1. Choose the next activity you've kept yourself from doing because of your weight, and make an active plan to begin doing it as soon as possible.

2. Repeat the previous steps by creating a mental movie trailer, affirmations, anchors, and dialoguing with your emotional self through your Inner Child Journal. This will empower you while using all of the other techniques as well to overcome any emotional obstacles or fears that get in your way.

3. Use the "Feel the Fear and Do it Anyway" Hypnotherapy Audio Session for each activity until you are no longer allowing your weight to hold you back from anything, and you live life fearlessly.

SUMMARY

Key Points

- Secondary gains are a neurosis in that they are designed to avoid anxiety and are often triggered by unresolved internal conflicts.

- Being overweight is often a way to avoid dealing with the true subconscious/conscious conflict between what you believe you consciously want, your negative core beliefs, and your subconscious/conscious fears that the negative core beliefs may be true. By staying overweight, you never have to do the things you say you want to do and risk failure.

- The fear of finding out that you may not be able to reach your goals because you don't *"have what it takes, aren't good enough, etc."* grows until you put an obstacle in your path that keeps you from having to face this fear of not being good enough. If you have struggled with life-long weight issues, being overweight is most likely this obstacle.

- When you begin doing the things you tell yourself you are going to do when you lose weight before you reach your weight loss goals, you eliminate excess body fat as an effective secondary gain. Since it is no longer working to hold you back anyway, your subconscious stops investing in it as a secondary gain and you stop self-sabotaging your weight loss efforts.

- You don't fully know if you have resolved your negative core beliefs until you're actively doing what you allowed these limiting beliefs to hold you back from doing.

- Feeling the fear and negative emotions related to moving forward with your goals, in spite of not having reached your desired level of weight loss, is normal. Using all of the tools you have learned in the *Fat to Fearless®* process so far, you can work through the anxiety and move forward anyway.

What This Has To Do With Weight Loss

If you have suffered from lifelong weight issues and are an emotional eater, being overweight has most likely become a way of protecting yourself from your fears of not being good enough or deficient in some way. Every time you come close to reaching your weight loss goals, the fear of doing and failing at the things you consciously say you will do when you lose weight causes you to subconsciously self-sabotage your dieting efforts. By doing these things before you reach your final weight loss goal, you can confront and overcome these fears before they interfere with your efforts to achieve the body you want.

You Are Ready To Move To The Next Chapter When . . .

- You have watched the tutorial video for this chapter (if you have the full *Fat to Fearless®* program).

- You have completed the exercises for this chapter in the Success Guide and Workbook (if you have the full *Fat to Fearless®* program).

CHAPTER 25

A FEARLESS LIFE

Congratulations on the hard work you've done through the *Fat to Fearless*® program. In the beginning, I told you that it wouldn't be easy, but it would be worth it. I'm sure you've found that to be true. If you've gone through the program, done all of the exercises while allowing yourself to be fully emotionally immersed in the process, while also listening to your Hypnotherapy Audio Sessions, then you understand why the only real permanent solution to weight loss is from the inside out. The *Fat to Fearless*® process isn't about loving yourself because you are thin, *but loving yourself enough to allow yourself to be thin!*

By now, you probably also uncovered the great secret of the *Fat to Fearless*® program, which is not simply a process to give you the tools to permanently end emotional eating and reach a healthy goal weight but also a methodology for allowing you to overcome any subconscious or emotional obstacles in your life. The ability to achieve any outcome is based on your ability to quiet your Inner Critic, empower yourself emotionally, take control of your thoughts, and move forward with solid action toward your goals while having the internal resources and skills to overcome any obstacles your own fears may put in your path.

In the beginning of the book you learned an important equation:

EVENTS → BELIEFS → EMOTIONS (resulting from experiences filtered through the beliefs) → SYMPTOMS → REINFORCE YOUR BELIEFS

This equation for how your negative core beliefs were formed and have led you into the Symptom Cycle that resulted in being overweight is something that you are intimately aware of now. However, in the beginning of the book I also promised you that everything that previously worked against you would be transformed to work for you, so it is now with this powerful equation.

Events

By making the conscious choice to live fearlessly and engage in activities that you want to avoid doing because you may not be at your final goal weight, you create new events that provide the opportunity to create new beliefs.

Beliefs

From these new events, new beliefs form around your self-worth and capabilities. When you apply all that you've learned to any negative thoughts, limiting beliefs, or uncomfortable feelings as they come up while engaging in these new events, you are able to consciously choose to reinforce your new beliefs. From living fearlessly, while using all that you've learned to address any limitations that come up for you during these events, you create new beliefs such as *"I am more than good enough, lovable, worthwhile, valuable, in control, etc."*

Emotions

Living life, filtering all of your new experiences through these new positive and life-affirming core beliefs, results in your feeling emotions. Happiness, pride, joy, satisfaction, bravery, love for self and others, and feeling empowered are just a few of the emotions that are likely to be a larger part of your daily experience.

Symptoms

While symptoms are technically defined as negative in nature, regardless of the term used, our emotional states drive behaviors. Previously, our negative emotions that emanated from our negative core beliefs produced symptoms of overeating and being overweight; now, however, your new positive beliefs and the resulting positive emotions produce different behaviors. You now find yourself living life more fully, not holding yourself back from the experiences in life you desire. Whether you have completely reached your goal weight or are in the process, you no longer use your weight to define your value and worth as a person.

Reinforce Your Beliefs

By engaging in these new activities through the lens of your new positive beliefs you provide tangible proof to both your conscious and subconscious that you are worthy, lovable, more than good enough, and deserve the best life has to offer. This only serves to positively reinforce your new beliefs while propelling you to expand your personal boundaries even further as you continue to spiral up.

As you can see by going from *Fat to Fearless®*, all that previously worked against you is now working for you. Should any difficulties arise along the way, you now have the tools to address them and continue moving forward while creating the life of your dreams.

It's also important to understand that human behavior isn't a constant. You are inextricably intertwined with your environment and those around you in a way that life is always presenting new challenges and obstacles. When these opportunities for growth arise, there is always a choice. You can either engage in old behavior patterns and ways of thinking that lead to mindless eating and self-destructive behavior, or you can apply all that you've learned to new situations that arise to ensure you rise above them and keep the body you worked so hard to achieve.

In the instances where I've seen people begin to backslide, which when specifically applied to the subject of this book means gaining weight, it's because of two things: First, is failing to understand that human behavior isn't black and white and there are no magical on and off buttons that mean we will never have problems again, and secondly not immediately applying the *Fat to Fearless*® lessons you've learned to yourself the moment you find yourself "backsliding." The moment you find yourself feeling the negative feelings that have driven you in the past to engage in unwanted behaviors is the same moment it is time to begin using the tools you now have by going through this process.

The types of changes you've created within yourself must be actively applied every day until they become automatic. Some days you will take two steps forward, and some days you may take half a step back. It's not that you will never be tempted again or ever briefly engage in unhealthy eating behaviors, it's that if it happens it's very seldom. When it does happen, you have the beliefs and tools that support you to get back on track. The challenge comes when you begin to think you simply do these exercises and learn these skills once, and then forget about them.

When you believe that you've simply flipped a switch and no longer need to actively apply what you've learned on an ongoing basis, then you're ill-prepared for times of temptation brought about by stressful situations or changes in lifestyle. Freedom isn't free is a phrase that also applies to living a fearless life with the body you want. The price of your freedom from diets and weight loss struggles is constant vigilance and application of all you've learned until it becomes second nature. The good news is that eventually it will become easy and automatic.

If you abandon your Inner Child, it will again begin to feel the negative emotions that make you want to reach for food. If you're not actively and continuously disassembling the lies of the Inner Critic, you'll soon find it becomes more negative again. If you're not making sure you have more pleasure than pain in your life, you may again find yourself reaching for a quick food fix. The good news is that the more time that goes by that you continuously apply what you've learned to your life, the easier and more automatic it becomes. Eventually, you almost unconsciously achieve self-mastery of your feelings and behaviors.

Failure isn't "never making a mistake or being tempted again." The beginning of failure is not recognizing that not always perfectly succeeding every time is part of the human experience. When it comes to weight loss and fitness you've probably heard it needs to be a "lifestyle change." I'm often asked what that means, and my response is that a lifestyle change is when more times than not you do the right things at the right times in the right ways, while building forward momentum that makes it continuously easier as time goes by. Your goal is a lifestyle change of continuously applying all you've learned as you move forward living life fearlessly.

Now that you've gone through the program once, I strongly suggest you start all over again. If you remember, in the beginning I explained how I had to take what was often a simultaneous process and put it into a linear format for the program and book. I also said that in live therapy many of these processes occur out of order and simultaneously, and once you complete the program and have the entire skill set to use as needed, you would begin making quantum leaps forward in your ability to enlist your subconscious mind and your emotions toward helping you reach your weight loss goals.

Almost everyone that has gone through the program a second time, having received a basic understanding from the first time through, has discovered they were able to get even more out of it and work at an even deeper level of transformation. The key to this program is not simply to read it and apply it once and put it on a shelf. As someone who went from living a life of fear in a prison of fat to living fearlessly in the body I always wanted, I can promise you everything I've taught you works to the degree that you continue to apply it. Like all things in life, the more you put into it the more you get out of it.

Another great way of using the program is to go through it again substituting 'weight loss' for any other area of life that you have repeatedly failed to achieve success despite a strong constant conscious desire to do so. Everything you've learned has universal application and, no matter what the goal you are actively working on, strengthening your relationship with your inner self while continuing to improve your ability to consciously choose your beliefs and behaviors will also continue to strength your ongoing abilities as they relate to food and weight loss.

My second suggestion for continued success is to stay involved in the *Fat to Fearless*® community to receive continued support and free updates. In live sessions I am able to determine the exact right combination of therapies to get the fastest results for each individual who sits in front of me. However, when I created this program, I had to decide what techniques and lessons to include that would be the most effective without making the book and program so large and complex that it might seem off-putting. Had I included all of the techniques I've created over the years to help people master weight loss, this book would easily be three times its size. My solution was to offer this program to you now, while providing you free program updates through my private social media community at www.asherfoxweightloss.org as well as my Facebook page www.facebook.com/asherfoxweightloss. If you haven't done so already, please go there now and register to be a part of an amazing group of people that are dedicated to coming together to lose weight, transform their lives, and live fearlessly.

Lastly, as part of the *Fat to Fearless®* community, you will receive information and techniques about my upcoming program: Weight Loss Willpower and Movement Motivation™. Whereas *Fat to Fearless®* has dealt with conquering the emotional aspects of weight loss, there may still be a lifetime of unhealthy habits that need to be replaced. Weight Loss Willpower and Movement Motivation™ deals with actually building conscious willpower by understanding the practical science of creating new healthy habits so that they become easy and automatic. While *Fat to Fearless®* has primarily focused on eliminating emotional eating and weight loss self-sabotage, this upcoming program will have a strong emphasis on learning to enjoy, and build habits around, exercise and movement while developing the ability to create motivation at will.

www.asherfoxweightloss.com/willpowerbook

It is my greatest desire that going through the *Fat to Fearless®* program has not only been educational and eye opening, but a transformational experience for you as well. It was for me and for the thousands of clients I've achieved success with. As I said in the beginning of the book, I'm now passing the baton to you to live the full, fearless, and happy life you've always wanted with the body you deserve to have. I would love to hear from you on your journey, so please email me at asher@asherfoxweightloss.com with any challenges you may have as well as your success stories as you go from *Fat to Fearless®*.

ADDITIONAL RESOURCES

The *Fat to Fearless*® program is designed to simulate, as closely as possible, personal sessions with myself using a combination of the book, Success Guide and Workbook, and Hypnotherapy Audio Sessions. The program does an amazing job of creating personal transformation as quickly as possible using media as opposed to live interactive sessions. That being said, for those interested in creating permanent change more quickly, I offer three other options as well.

Live *Fat to Fearless*® sessions with me in my Orlando, FL, office involve a combination of all of the techniques in this book holistically applied to your specific psyche, goals, and life situation. There are some very powerful techniques that you can't do alone that can produce almost instantly the same results as months of work on your own. In addition to Orlando residents, I also offer 2 and 3-day private programs for those who wish to experience the power of rapid change. More information about the techniques I use in these sessions as well as Frequently Asked Questions can be found at:

www.asherfoxweightloss.com/orlandosessions

Live *Fat to Fearless*® Skype sessions with me allow us to work together to uncover your hidden core beliefs, create customized Hypnotherapy Audio Sessions specifically for your goals, as well as actively work through the program to overcome your specific set of challenges. More information about Skype sessions with me can be found at:

www.asherfoxweightloss.com/onlinesessions

Live *Fat to Fearless*® online or telephone group sessions allow you to get personalized attention with built-in support from others who are also going through the process. Group coaching is either on the phone or online and includes recordings of all group sessions as well as additional bonus materials. More information about group coaching sessions with me can be found at:

www.asherfoxweightloss.com/groupcoaching

BIBLIOGRAPHY

Asher is an expert in the synthesis of varying therapeutic schools of thought and fields of study into comprehensive, effective, and practical approaches to rapidly healing psychological and emotional issues. The notes listed below refer to sources used in the development of much of the material in the *Fat to Fearless*® program.

John Bradshaw, *Homecoming: Reclaiming and Championing Your Inner Child*, (USA: Bantam, 1990).

Gil Boyne, *Transforming Therapy: A New Approach to Hypnotherapy*, (USA: Westwood Publishing company, Inc., 1985).

Josie Hadley & Carol Staudacher, *Hypnosis for Change*, (USA: New Harbinger Publications, 1996).

John G. Kappas, Ph.D., *Professional Hypnotism Manual, Rev. Ed 2009*, (USA: Panorama Publishing Company, 2009).

Patrick Fanning, *Visualization for Change, 2nd Edition*, (USA: New Harbinger Publications, 1994).

Richard Bandler & John Grinder, *Trance-Formations*, (USA: Real People Press, 1981).

Dave Elman, *Hypnotherapy*, (USA: Westwood Publishing company, Inc., 1964).

Shakti Gawain, *Creative Visualization*, (USA: Nataraj Publishing, 1978).

Tim Simmerman, *Medical Hypnotherapy, Volume One*, (USA: Peaceful Planet Press, 2007).

Dan Baker, Ph.D. & Cameron Stauth, *What Happy People Know*, (USA: St. Martin's Griffin, 2004).

Richard Bandler & John Grinder, *Frogs into Princes*, (USA: Real People Press, 1979).

Richard Bandler & John Grinder, *Structure of Magic,* (USA: Science and Behavior Books Inc., 1975).

Robert Dilts, *Changing Belief Systems with NLP*, (USA: Meta Publications, 1990).

Neville, *The Power of Awareness,* (USA: Start Publishing LLC, 2012).

Leonard Mlodinow, *How Your Unconscious Mind Rules Your Behavior*, (USA: Pantheon Books, 2012).

Les Fehmi, Ph.D. & Jim Robbins, *The Open-Focus Brain* (USA: Trumpeter Books, 2007).

David Eagleman, *Incognito, The Secret Lives of the Brain*, (USA: Pantheon Books, 2011).

John Assaraf & Murray Smith, *The Answer*, (USA: Atria Books, 2008).

L.P. Midler, *Erik H. Erikson and Intimacy vs. Isolation*, (USA: Critical Mass Publications, 2012).

Dilts, Griner, Bandler & Delozier, *NLP, Volume 1*, (USA: Meta Publications, 1980).

C.G. Jung, *Collected Works of C.G. Jung, Volume 9 (part1) 2nd Edition: Archetypes and the Collective Unconscious*, (USA: Princeton University Press, 2014).

Dawson Church, Ph.D., *The EFT Manual, Third Edition*, (USA: Energy Psychology Press, 2013).

Eric Berne, M.D., *Games People Play*, (USA: Ballantine Books, 1996).

Richard Bandler & John Grinder, *Patterns of the Hypnotic Techniques of Milton H. Erickson, M.D. Volume 1*, (USA: Meta Publications, 1975).

www.ingramcontent.com/pod-product-compliance
Lightning Source LLC
Chambersburg PA
CBHW060834280326
41934CB00007B/772